# SURGICAL TRANSCRIPTIONS AND PEARLS IN OBSTETRICS AND GYNECOLOGY

# SURGICAL TRANSCRIPTIONS AND PEARLS IN OBSTETRICS AND GYNECOLOGY

## Second Edition

### John E Turrentine MD

*Hamilton Medical Center*
*Dalton, GA, USA*

### Forewords written by

### Neal H Newsom MD

*Associate Clinical Instructor*
*Department of Gynecology and Obstetrics*
*Emory University School of Medicine*
*Atlanta, GA, USA*

### and

### Lindsay R Fields MD

*Medical College of Georgia*
*Augusta, GA, USA*

## informa
healthcare

© 1994, 2006 Informa UK Ltd

First published in the United Kingdom in 1994
By The Parthenon Publishing Group

Second edition published in 2006
by Informa UK Ltd, 4 Park Square, Milton Park, Abingdon, Oxon OX14 4RN

Tel: +44 (0)20 7017 6000
Fax: +44 (0)20 7017 6699
E-mail: info.medicine@tandf.co.uk
Website: www.tandf.co.uk/medicine

A CIP record for this book is available from the British Library.

Library of Congress Cataloging-in-Publication Data

Data available on application

ISBN10 0 415 39770 7
ISBN13 978 0 415 39770 4

Distributed in North and South America by
Taylor & Francis
6000 Broken Sound Parkway, NW, (Suite 300)
Boca Raton, FL 33487, USA

*Within Continental USA*
Tel: 1(800) 272 7737; Fax: 1(800) 374 3401
*Outside Continental USA*
Tel: (561) 994 0555; Fax: (561) 361 6018
E-mail: *orders@crcpress.com*

Distributed in the rest of the world by
Thomson Publishing Services
Cheriton House
North Way
Andover, Hampshire SP10 5BE, UK
Tel: +44 (0)1264 332424
E-mail: tps.tandfsalesorder@thomson.com

Composition by J&L Composition, Filey, North Yorkshire
Printed and bound in Spain by Grafos SA Arte Sobre Papel

Thanks to my sons, Jake and Joe,
for their help with the editing process.

# Contents

# Foreword

The concept of a compilation of dictated operative reports and conversion of them into book form is intriguing and unique. To the best of my knowledge, it has not been done before, and is one of those things that makes you wonder 'Why didn't I think of doing that before now?'

Most of our medical expertise develops from clinical, on-the-job training with 'hands on' patient care, and no book, monograph, or journal article to guide your hand to ensure that you become a master craftsman, with the technique and skill required to perform proficient surgery. These come from experience in the operating room, under proper tutelage. This publication, however, may serve as a wonderful reference and guideline for the neophyte who needs a description of the game plan. It may also be of value to the more experienced surgeon – as a refresher, from time to time. How many of us have re-read our own old Op Notes on cases that we do not perform very often? If you have not, maybe you should.

I remember an old saying from my residency program: see one – do one – teach one. This is a catchy phrase, but, in this day and time, totally inadequate. I would offer: scrub on a dozen, do a hundred, then teach. And teaching should be from a true desire and willingness to impart our art and knowledge to our fledgling members and professional colleagues, rather than, perhaps, some other less honorable motivations. Hopefully, this book will do just that, and be a helpful adjunct and catalyst in the quest for excellent patient care.

I have personally known Johnny Turrentine since his childhood, as a next-door neighbor, and then as a professional colleague at the same hospital for several years. He is a fine gentleman in all matters, and I wish him good fortune and contentment in the fulfillment of his life's dream.

**Neal H Newsom MD**
Associate Clinical Instructor
Department of Gynecology and Obstetrics
Emory University School of Medicine
Atlanta, GA
USA

# Foreword

I first met Dr Turrentine during my third year clinical clerkship in obstetrics and gynecology. I had scheduled obstetrics and gynecology as my first rotation, as I had little interest in the field and considered myself a future pediatrician. By the end of the first week my career plans had changed. I was truly amazed by Dr Turrentine's enthusiasm toward his work, his dedication to his patients, and his meticulous surgical technique. His enthusiasm was contagious, and I knew that I too, was destined for a career in obstetrics and gynecology. I've never looked back.

Dr Turrentine has been such an inspiration to me. During the six weeks of my clerkship, I assisted him with the surgery he developed, the MIVH (minimally invasive vaginal hysterectomy). I watched these women as they recovered from surgery and walked out of the hospital, smiling, in less than a day. I later found out from my classmates that women often take weeks to recover from the more traditional abdominal or vaginal approaches. I consider the MIVH as only one of many things that Dr Turrentine has done for others. By creating shorter hospital stays for his patients, by helping me excel on my obstetrics and gynecology shelf exam, or by writing this new book for residents and surgeons, Dr Turrentine always seems to be doing everything he can to help others. Truly, he is an inspiring man.

The second edition of *Surgical Transcriptions and Pearls in Obstetrics and Gynecology* is a wonderful compilation of transcriptions and clinical wisdom that will be incredibly helpful for any new obstetrics and gynecology student. As I will begin my obstetrics and gynecology residency in less than six months, I am very grateful to know about this publication! I plan to use this book as a tool to better prepare myself for cases, and I trust that I will feel much more confident when the scalpel is in my hand. Thanks so much to Dr Turrentine – excellent surgeon, physician, teacher, and friend.

**Lindsay R Fields MD**
4th year Medical Student
Medical College of Georgia
Augusta, GA
USA

# Abbreviations

| | |
|---|---|
| ABG | Arterial blood gas |
| ACOG | American College of Obstetricians and Gynecologists |
| AIVS | Anterior intravaginal sling |
| A&P REPAIR | Anterior and posterior repair (colporrhaphy) |
| AROM | Augmented rupture of membranes |
| BSO | Bilateral salpingo-oophorectomy (removal of both tubes and ovaries) |
| C/S | Cesarean section |
| D & E or D & C | Dilatation and evacuation (or) dilatation and curettage |
| DIC | Disseminated intravascular coagulation |
| DUB | Dysfunctional uterine bleeding |
| EBL | Estimated blood loss |
| ERT | Estrogen replacement therapy |
| EUA | Examination under anesthesia |
| EXP. LAP | Exploratory laparotomy |
| GNH | German needle holder |
| GSI | Genuine stress incontinence |
| HALSH | Hand-assisted laparoscopic surgical hysterectomy |
| HRT | Hormone replacement therapy |
| IPG | Implantable pulse generator |
| IUP | Intrauterine pressure |
| IVP | Intravenous pyelogram |
| LAVH | Laparoscopic-assisted vaginal hysterectomy |
| LEEP | Loop electrocoagulation excision procedure |
| LFD | Low forcep delivery |
| LOA | Left occipitant anterior |
| LOP | Left occipitant posterior |

| | |
|---|---|
| LOT | Left occipitant transverse |
| LSH | Laparoscopic supracervical hysterectomy |
| LSO | Left salpingo-oophorectomy (removal of left tube and ovary) |
| LUNA | Laparoscopic uterosacral nerve ablation |
| MAC | Monitored anesthesia care |
| MFD | Mid-forcep delivery |
| MIVH | Minimally invasive vaginal hysterectomy |
| MMK | Marshall–Marchetti–Krantz procedure |
| Monsel's | Ferrous subsulfate solution |
| OA | Occipitant anterior |
| OP | Occipitant posterior |
| OT | Occipitant transverse |
| PACU | Post anesthesia care unit |
| PID | Pelvic inflammatory disease |
| PIVS | Posterior intravaginal sling |
| PONV | Post-op nausea and vomiting |
| ROA | Right occipitant anterior |
| ROP | Right occipitant posterior |
| ROT | Right occipitant transverse |
| RSO | Right salpingo-oophorectomy (removal of right tube and ovary) |
| RX | Treatment |
| SCOPE | Laparoscopy (or) videolaparoscopy |
| SPROM | Spontaneous premature rupture of membranes |
| SPROM NIL | Spontaneous premature rupture of membranes not in labor |
| SRNH | Self-righting needle holder |
| SROM | Spontaneous rupture of membranes |
| SUI | Stress urinary incontinence |
| SVD | Spontaneous vaginal delivery |
| TAH | Total abdominal hysterectomy |

| | |
|---|---|
| TLH | Total laparoscopic hysterectomy |
| TOA | Tubo-ovarian abscess |
| TOT | Transobturator tape |
| TSH | Total supracervical hysterectomy |
| TVH | Total vaginal hysterectomy |
| TVT | Tension-free vaginal tape |
| VAIN | Vaginal intraepithelial neoplasia |
| VBAC | Vaginal birth after C-section |
| VBG | Venous blood gas |
| VE | Vacuum extraction |
| VLL | Video laser laparoscopy |

# Introduction

Dr Turrentine spent several years developing, writing, and updating the *Surgical Transcription in Obstetrics and Gynecology*. Dr Turrentine indicated that when he was 'going through' the gauntlet of medical school externships, internship, and residency, he found himself learning how to actually perform surgery by reading about the procedure prior to the surgery and then transcribing the surgery. At the time he transcribed the surgery, he would often use an experienced physician's transcription of a similar case as a guide. He would change his dictation as to how the procedure was actually done. He would again read the textbook to make certain he had included all the information necessary for proper documentation. This method was quite tedious. Dr Turrentine always wondered why no one would just research and write a manual of common surgical procedures to use as a guide. Many of his peers also felt a manual would be helpful. Dr Turrentine has also seen many changes in surgical technology over the past 20 years. One has to stay abreast of these changes; hence, the reason for this second edition. However, rather than just an update of the first edition, Dr Turrentine thought it best to also include more pearls of surgery and thus rename the second edition as *Surgical Transcriptions and Pearls in Obstetrics and Gynecology*.

Dr Turrentine received his medical degree from the Medical College of Georgia in Augusta, Georgia and received a Doctor of Ministry from Trinity Seminary (Liverpool, England). He completed an obstetrics and gynecology internship at the University of Southern California/Los Angeles County Women's Hospital and completed his residency at Atlanta Medical Center. He then spent several years in practice with his father, who had 44 years of obstetrics and gynecology experience. Dr Turrentine worked and lectured with the laparoscopic physicians Saye, McCarus, and Nezhat during the 'birth' of this technique. He also spent many hours with the late Cullen Richardson, learning as much as possible about pelvic reconstruction and vaginal surgery. He moved with his family from the 'big city' to a 'small town'. His rural practice in the 'trenches' provided him with the pleasant surprise of up-to-date technology and an extensive high-volume clinical experience. Dr Turrentine performed 35–40 gynecological cases and approximately 30 obstetric cases per month for many years. He delivered triplets and numerous twins, including two sets just moments apart. He faced many high-risk situations without the cushion of subspecialists. He had to perform many procedures, including emergencies without anesthesia coverage or surgical back-up. After 10 years of solo practice in Northwestern North Carolina and then building a four-doctor practice over the next 2 years, he sold his practice and moved back to Georgia. He became a Clinical Professor for the Medical College of Georgia and Director of Surgical Technology at Dalton

State College. Dr Turrentine is a Board Certified Diplomate and Fellow of the American College of Obstetricians and Gynecologists. He also trained with Niall Galloway at Emory School of Medicine, learning as much about urogynecology as possible. He became certified in periurethral injections and pelvic reconstruction and urogynecological surgery. He then became a preceptor for Bard Surgical, Inc. and Ethicon Endo-Surgical, Inc. He presently teaches advanced urological, laparoscopic, and advanced minimally invasive vaginal procedures throughout the country. He also lectures at many Grand Rounds and medical meetings throughout the USA and Europe. Dr Turrentine developed, named, and now teaches MIVH (minimally invasive vaginal hysterectomy). He continues to remain busy in clinical practice, in obstetrics, obstetric anesthesia, and gynecological surgery. He maintains an Ob/Gyn solo practice in Northwest Georgia. Many changes and advances in surgical procedures have occurred since Dr Turrentine authored his original *Surgical Transcription in Obstetrics and Gynecology*. Therefore, on examining this book, the reader will know that Dr Turrentine's continued experience and training qualifies him to revise and update his original very 'clinical' manual.

It is important for interns, residents, and even clinical practitioners to be able to learn a type of 'form dictation' following their operations. Although every surgical operation is different, this book certainly does not include the complications and unexpected findings so often encountered. The book has been researched carefully using standard academic textbooks and recent articles. Combined with Dr Turrentine's extensive clinical experience, it should enable the obstetrician/gynecologist to use this book as both a learning protocol and a guide to transcriptions for common obstetric and gynecological procedures. Many of the recommended transcriptions may be Dr Turrentine's preference and should not be considered the medicolegal standard of care. Many institutions may not be equipped with the technology described in this book. The book, however, is excellent for the beginning surgeon and can also be used by the experienced but tired obstetrics and gynecological specialist who might be dictating his operation in the middle of the night. These physicians would certainly not want inadvertently to omit some important aspect of their surgery that they automatically perform from years of training. This book should not necessarily dictate the exact form that should be transcribed but would certainly make an excellent guide to all obstetrical and gynecological physicians during their postsurgical transcriptions. This book should be important not only for more accurate medical record-keeping but also for reducing the medicolegal risks. It also includes many of the newer technologies and equipment along with pearls in regard to the advantages and disadvantages of certain types of instruments.

These surgical transcriptions should be read before using the contents of this book. There will be variation in surgical techniques from surgeon to surgeon. The importance of using this book solely as a guide should be highlighted to all obstetricians/gynecologists.

Many hospitals and institutions throughout the country have developed a number of suggestions and recommendations as regards to the methods of communication and 'how to' proceed with suitable dictations. There are very wide variations from institution to institution and each is generally a reflection of each hospital's recommendation. Many Medical Record Committees have come up with a number of suggestions that have been implemented at hospitals throughout the nation. When dictating an operative note, the typical format is:

(1) Date of dictation
(2) Date of surgery
(3) Name of patient
(4) Hospital medical record number of patient
(5) Pre-op diagnosis
(6) Post-op diagnosis
(7) Operation (name of procedure)
(8) Indications for surgery
(9) Pathology or findings at time of surgery
(10) Surgeon
(11) Assistant(s)
(12) Anesthesia
(13) Anesthesiologist(s)/anesthetist(s),
(14) Explanation of the procedure (technique)
(15) Estimated blood loss
(16) Fluid or blood replacement (if any or if significant)
(17) Condition of patient on arrival at recovery room.

This book will contain numbers 7 and 14 in regard to the sample transcriptions, as these are the dictations that will remain fairly consistent.

The following explanations and sample transcription should be of help to any beginning intern or resident in obstetrics and gynecology who needs to be reassured that he is keeping up with the safety features, technology, and improved methods of performing and transcribing obstetrics and gynecology procedures.

There will be three sample transcriptions of Dr Turrentine's surgeries taken directly from actual cases. Form transcriptions will then follow and can be easily found in alphabetical order in the table of contents with special sections for certain types of surgery. There is also included an overview on some of the major categories and important points where Dr Turrentine thought they would be helpful for the surgeon learning the procedure. Dr Turrentine hopes this will be as helpful to the Ob/Gyn surgeon as he wished it had been available to him.

# Sample transcriptions

The following are three full sample transcriptions. These procedures were performed prior to 1991. Since that time, many of the techniques have changed. C-sections are even performed differently. Some practitioners do not even close the bladder, peritoneum, and/or adipose tissue. Some only close the uterus in one layer. In laparoscopic cases, many surgeons have abandoned the Verres needle and use the Hasson (open technique). Laparoscopic cases, such as the one below, now include using either the Cryomyomectomy technique to freeze the fibroid or the liberal use of suturing techniques. However, these samples are retained to show how only 10–15 years of surgery can change so drastically. The book will guide the gynecological surgeon through the step-by-step process of the cutting edge of modern surgery. The remainder of transcriptions in this book include names and techniques only, with pearls from experience where I felt necessary.

**SAMPLE 1**

Hugh Chatham Memorial Hospital

OPERATIVE PROCEDURE

| Name | Number | Sex | Age |
|------|--------|-----|-----|
| ************* | ****** | F | 25 |

| Admit | Disc. | Med. Record# | Type | Room# |
|-------|-------|--------------|------|-------|
| ****** | ***** | ****** | O/P | 357 |

Date of Birth   8/17/1966                    _____ Physician _____
Physician   4201 TURRENTINE JOHN
**Surgeon**   Dr TURRENTINE                **Assistant**
**Date**

**Preoperative Diagnosis:**        Incomplete spontaneous abortion

**Postoperative Diagnosis:**       Same

**Procedure:**                     Suction dilatation and evacuation

**Anesthesia**:                    General

**Anesthetist**:                   Foster, CRNA

**Findings:** The uterus was approximately 9 weeks' size. The cervix was already dilated with tissue and blood oozing from the cervical os.

**Technique:** Patient was prepped and draped in the usual manner for a vaginal procedure. Weighted speculum was placed into the vagina and a Sims retractor was used on the anterior portion of the vagina. A single tooth tenaculum was attached to the anterior lip of the cervix and the cervix was already noted to be dilated and enabled a #31 Pratt dilator to be admitted. Bleeding was very brisk and there was tissue protruding from the cervix. Using a #8 curved suction tip the intrauterine cavity was systematically emptied using the suction evacuation apparatus. After the intrauterine cavity was felt to be smooth and empty, a light sharp curette was utilized on the intrauterine cavity. Bleeding seemed to be decreased and the suction tip was again used on the intrauterine cavity. Hemostasis appeared to be excellent and a 4 × 4 sponge was held against the cervix for approximately 45 seconds after the intrauterine cavity had felt to be smooth and empty. The patient tolerated the procedure very well and all instrumentation was removed from the vagina.

John Turrentine, MD/mt
D: 6-23-92   T: 6-23-92

**SAMPLE 2**

## Hugh Chatham Memorial Hospital

### OPERATIVE PROCEDURE

| **Name** | **Number** | Sex | Age |
|---|---|---|---|
| ************* | ****** | F | 25 |

| Admit | Disc. | **Med. Record#** | Type | Room# |
|---|---|---|---|---|
| ****** | ***** | ****** | I/P | 362 |

Date of Birth   6/08/1967                    _____ Physician _____
Physician   4201 TURRENTINE JOHN
**Surgeon**   Dr TURRENTINE                **First Assistant**   Dr Peterson
Pediatricians   Dr Erlandson, Dr Groner, Dr Stuart
**Date**

**Preoperative Diagnosis:**
1. Borderline preterm labor
2. PIH with HELLP syndrome
3. Triplet, multiple gestation
4. Primip breech baby C presentation

**Postoperative Diagnosis:**   Same

**Procedure:**   Primary Kerr Cesarean section

**Anesthetist:**   Roger Gates

**Anesthesia:**   Epidural (Jet)

Infant Statistics
Baby A: sex female, presentation vertex, weight 4 pounds 10.6 ounces, apgars 8 and 10, umbilical cord blood gas ABG 7.25, VBG 7.29.

Baby B: sex female, presentation vertex, weight 3 pounds 12 ounces, apgars 7 and 9, umbilical cord blood gas ABG 7.20, VBG 7.17.

Baby C: sex female, presentation breech, weight 4 pounds 15 ounces, apgars 7 and 8, umbilical cord blood gas ABG 7.33, VBG 7.33.

Estimated Blood Loss: 600 ml

**Technique:** Patient was prepped and draped in the usual manner for a low Pfannenstiel abdominal incision. Incision was carried down through the subcutaneous tissue of the fascia. The fascia was incised with scalpel blade and extended in a smiling fashion by sharp dissection using the Mayo scissors. Overlying muscle tissue was sharply dissected away from the overlying fascia. The peritoneum was entered with sharp dissection using the Metzenbaum scissors and two hemostats to lift the entry site away from the underlying abdominal viscera. The bladder was then sharply dissected away from the lower uterine segment using smooth forceps and Metzenbaum scissors. The bladder flap retractor was then placed between the uterus and bladder to expose the lower uterine segment.

The incision was carried out using the scalpel and entry into the uterus was made, being careful to expose the amniotic sac. The amniotic sac was entered and fluid was noted to be clear and there was no foul odor. Extension of the incision into the uterus was carried out in a low transverse smiling fashion, being careful to avoid major vasculature along the lower uterine segment bilaterally. Baby A's head was lifted into view so as to expose the scalp in order to place the vacuum extractor. A pressure of 580 mmHg was applied in order to bring the head out of the uterus and, with gentle pressure, the remainder of the baby was removed from the uterus. The outer glove of the right hand, which had been in the lower uterine segment, was removed and the baby's oropharynx was suctioned thoroughly with the suction bulb. The umbilical cord was clamped in sections for cord blood gas analysis, routine blood testing, and immediate complete blood count (stat CBC) to rule out twin-twin transfusion. Baby A cord was identified by one clamp at the end of the umbilical cord. The section closest to the infant was cut with scissors beyond the cord clamp and between the first clamp across the cord, and then the infant was removed from the operative field by Dr Stuart. The infant was spontaneously crying. The second amniotic sac was easily visible and this was ruptured with an Allis clamp and found to be clear and without an odor. The head easily came into view and the vacuum extraction was placed on this baby's head and easily extracted. The remainder of the baby was delivered and the infant was spontaneously crying as the oropharynx was suctioned thoroughly with the suction bulb. An umbilical clamp was placed on the umbilical cord and then two clamps were placed immediately distal to the umbilical cord clamp for identification of umbilical cord B and then two sections of cord were clamped apart from this for cord pH, routine blood testing, and stat CBC. The cord was cut between the umbilical cord clamp and the two clamps and the baby was removed from the operative field by Dr Groner. Debbie Myers RN. was working with Dr Groner and Luann Brooks RN. was working with Dr Stuart with Baby A. The third amniotic sac was located and ruptured with the Allis clamp. The fluid was noted to be slightly meconium stained. There was no foul odor. The infant was noted to be in a double footling breech presentation and an attempt at location of the fetal parts was performed for possible internal version but, because of the small size of the baby and difficulty in location of placenta and multiple cords, it was decided that the best maneuver to deliver the baby would be by breech extraction. The two legs were grasped and in a corkscrew fashion the remainder of the infant was delivered until the shoulders were consecutively delivered. Using the Mauriceau maneuver the infant's head was delivered and it was crying spontaneously even prior to suctioning. Suctioning was performed, however, and then the cords were clamped with an umbilical cord clamp and three clamps just distal to the umbilical cord clamp and then the cord was clamped into sections for routine blood testing, cord pH, and stat CBC. The infant was removed from the operative field by Dr Erlandson, being assisted by Sandra Luffman RN. Multiple umbilical cords were easily identified by the one, two, and three clamps and the placentas were then removed; it was found that baby A and B shared a placenta and baby C was contained in a separate placental unit.

Following removal of the two large placentas, the patient was given several ampules of pitocin and the uterus was also injected with PGF-2 alpha to reduce the uterine size and decrease the chance of uterine atony. The patient was also given 3 g of Unasyn IV. The intrauterine cavity was checked very carefully for any remaining products of conception and, having made certain that there was none, the uterine incision was reapproximated in two layers. The first layer was closed in an interlocking continuous 0 chromic suture. The second layer was approximated over the first layer using a continuous limbered style 0 chromic suture. Hemostasis was excellent and the bladder was then reapproximated with 2-0 chromic continuous suture. After the uterus and adnexa were in the proper anatomical position in the pelvis, the uterus was inspected again and found to be very firm and there was no need for any further treatment for possible uterine atony. The abdomen was inspected and found to be in normal appearance, including the appendix. The peritoneum was closed in a continuous fashion, 0 delayed absorbable suture incorporating the rectus muscle simultaneously. The fascia was reapproximated with 2-0 Vicryl in a continuous fashion. The subcutaneous tissue was closed with 3-0 plain on a large needle. Skin was reapproximated with 5-0 Vicryl in a subcuticular fashion. The incision was wiped clean with wet lap dry lap and benzoin was applied. Steri-strips were applied over the incision and then bandage was applied. Sponge, lap, instrument, and needle counts were all correct. The patient was given Duramorph epidurally and moved to the Recovery Room in good condition. The triplets were also in stable condition.

John E Turrentine, MD/pbg
D:   12-5-92
T:   12-7-92
cc:  Dr Peterson
     Dr Stuart
     Dr Erlandson

**SAMPLE 3**

Hamilton Medical Center
Dalton, Georgia

OPERATIVE PROCEDURE

| **Name** | **Number** | Sex | Age |
|---|---|---|---|
| ************* | ****** | F | 24 |

| Admit | Disc. | **Med. Record#** | Type | Room# |
|---|---|---|---|---|
| ****** | ***** | ****** | O/P | 357 |

Date of Birth   8/18/1968 _____ Physician _____
Physician   4201 TURRENTINE JOHN
**Surgeon**   Dr TURRENTINE
**Date**

**Preoperative Diagnosis:**   Uterine fibroids with pelvic pain and infertility

**Postoperative Diagnosis:**   Same

**Anesthesia:**   General

**Anesthesiologist:**   Dr Justice

**Procedure:** Diagnostic fractional D & C with videolaparoscopic multiple myomectomies

**Findings:** There were two fibroids. One very large anterior fundal fibroid approximately 7 cm in diameter. This was on a thick stalk. There was a second smaller 12–14 mm subserosal fibroid along the right side of the uterus.

**Technique:** The patient was prepped and draped with Betadine solution and draped in the lithotomy position with special attention to the area of the umbilicus and cervix. Weighted speculum was placed into the vagina so as to expose the cervix. A single-toothed tenaculum was placed on the anterior lip of the cervix and ECC was obtained in routine manner. Dilators (Pratt) were used until the cervix was dilated enough to allow entrance of a light, sharp curette. Intrauterine cavity was curetted in the routine fashion, until endometrial curettings were obtained on Telfa pad. These were passed off to be sent to Pathology. There was no fatty or unusual tissue noted. A single-toothed tenaculum was replaced with a uterine manipulator. The weighted speculum was removed from the vagina and the bladder was emptied with a red rubber catheter. Gloves were changed prior to the abdominal incision.

A small subumbilical incision was performed, and a Surgiport Verres needle was placed in the incision and checked by the syringe, hanging drop, bubble and gas pressure register methods. All methods indicated proper placement of the needle. Pneumoperitoneum of approximately 3 liters of $CO_2$ was established and the Surgiport trocar was properly inserted in the abdomen. The sound of escaping gas confirmed proper location in the abdomen as the trocar was removed from the sleeve.

Videofiberoptics were connected to the laparoscope, and this was inserted through the 10 mm sleeve under videolaparoscopic visualization. Trendelenburg position was increased and approximately 1–1.5 liters more $CO_2$ was allowed into the abdomen to better displace the viscera so as to easily visualize the pelvic organs. There was noted a large fundal fibroid along the anterior portion of the uterine corpus, and another subserosal fibroid along the right cornual area near the entrance of the fallopian tube. It was at this point that a second trocar was placed. A 12 mm trocar was placed approximately 5–6 cm below the umbilical incision, and through the 10 mm sleeve the stalk was grasped with flat duckbill bipolar forceps and carefully coagulated from all sides for approximately 30 seconds until hemostasis was thought to be assured. The myoma was then excised with laparoscopic hook scissors. Oozing was controlled with the flat duckbill bipolar coagulator.

The myoma was then placed into the posterior cul-de-sac with four-prong graspers and then thorough irrigation was performed over the uterine fundus.

The embedded myoma was estimated as to size and extent, and it was decided that there was no need for any vasopressin injection because it was felt that the fibroid could be removed using the flat duckbill bipolar forceps and/or point coagulator. The coagulation was performed along the outside of the serosa.

The fibroid had to be manipulated through the single puncture until the stalk was reached and coagulation was performed using the flat duckbill bipolar forceps. Once the myoma was noted to be white due to ischemia, the serosal capsule was then endocoagulated with flat duckbill bipolar forceps, and the capsule was easily dissected away using the flat duckbill bipolar forceps, establishing a clean plane. After the capsule was systematically stripped off the myoma using the coagulator, the myoma was stabilized with large four-prong grasping forceps and further dissection was performed with the flat duckbill bipolar forceps and then the base was reached and care was taken not to lacerate any feeding vessels. Nevertheless, there was still some bleeding which was unable to be controlled with simply the flat duckbill bipolar forceps. The pedicle was able to be cut with the hook scissors and removed, and then hemostasis was brought into effect by placing the laparoscopic flat duckbill bipolar forceps into the bed where the fibroid had been removed. The myoma was detached by twisting the pedicle with the four-prong grasper as the base of the fibroid was being coagulated with the flat duckbill bipolar forceps. The four-prong grasper was then used to place the smaller fibroid into the posterior cul-de-sac.

The crater was then thoroughly irrigated with normal saline and inspected for hemostasis. Interceed was placed over both the cornual crater and over the fundal crater. Extraction was then attempted by using the four-prong grasper and pulling it up through the 12 mm trocar, but neither fibroid would be removed using this method. A posterior colpotomy was performed after several attempts to split the fibroids. A speculum was placed into the vagina. Retractors were utilized and an incision was made in the posterior vaginal wall and the peritoneum. Immediately the pneumoperitoneum was lost, and also the fibroids were lost. Videolaparoscopy could not be used to see the fibroids; therefore, my hand was placed into the pelvis through the posterior colpotomy, and the fibroids were palpated. An Allis clamp was then placed between my fingers, and the larger fibroid was extracted, but the smaller fibroid could not be reached. At this point the colpotomy incision was reapproximated and hemostasis was brought into effect using inter-rupted interlocking sutures of 0 chromic suture. Hemostasis was excellent, and pneumoperitoneum was again obtained.

Changing gloves, attention was then directed back into the abdomen with liberal use of Mandol/normal saline solution throughout the posterior cul-de-sac and pelvis. The patient had also been given Unasyn 3 grams approx-imately 20–30 minutes prior to making the vaginal incision. The smaller fibroid was then grasped and the irrigation was thoroughly removed from the pelvis – the pelvis appeared to be uninjured in regard to bowel, vessel, bladder, or ureter; the small fibroid was brought rapidly through the 12 mm sleeve as the sleeve was removed. With fibroid trapped between the fascia and sub-cutaneous layer, it was then grasped with a towel clip and removed from the lower incision. After assessing that hemostasis was excellent again, and that no injury had occurred to other structures, the pneumoperitoneum was again released, and instrumentation was removed under direct video visual-ization. Reapproximation of the incision was performed with interrupted suture of 2-0 delayed absorbable suture and placement of steri-strips and bandage was applied. Vaginal instrumentation was then removed, and hemostasis was considered excellent in the vaginal area too.

The patient went to the Recovery Room in good condition.

John E Turrentine, MD/lc
D:   11-17-92
T:   11-25-92

# Appendectomy

## Technique

The appendix was delivered into the operative field by rotation of the cecum up and out. The vessels within the mesoappendix were doubly ligated with _____ suture and then transected, with particular attention directed toward the appendicular artery.

A hemostat was applied to crush the base of the appendix. The hemostat was then moved distal so that another small clamp could be placed just below the resulting groove. *(The stump of the appendix may or may not be tied with a ligature in this groove.)*

The scalpel was used to amputate the appendix along the groove. The stump was then inverted into the cecum using the hemostat that had been placed below the groove. This stump was then buried under a purse-string suture of 3-0 _____ (silk) suture that had been placed through the seromuscular layers of the cecum.

The entire operative field around the appendiceal stump site was then irrigated with _____ (kanamycin, neomycin, or cefamandole solution). *(The tagged sutures of the mesoappendix can then optionally be tied into purse-string suture already closed.)*

(Describe the remainder of the closure.)

## Author's notes

Often, the appendix is removed during ovarian cancer staging, C-section, or hysterectomy. Many times, during surgery, prophylactic appendectomy may be done if fecaliths are found. Therefore, the benefits and arguments for and against McBurney incisions, paramedian incisions, drains, and other subjects associated with actual pathological findings will be omitted here. Technique of incidental appendectomy is described after already inside the peritoneum.

Incidental/non-emergent indications for appendectomy include:

(1) female 10–30 years of age
(2) female with exploratory surgery for unexplained pain
(3) female with exploratory surgery for RLQ (right lower quadrant) pain
(4) female who is mentally handicapped.

Contraindications for appendectomy include:

(1)  female with Crohn's disease
(2)  female with inaccessible appendix
(3)  presence of grafts or material
(4)  prior history of radiation
(5)  unstable medical condition.

# Bartholin's gland excision

### Technique

After the patient arrived in the Operating Room she was prepped and draped in the usual manner for a vaginal procedure. After proper prepping and draping, the Bartholin's duct cyst was located and an elliptical incision in the vaginal mucosa was made as close as possible to the site of the gland orifice. This incision was made on the mucosal side. Utilizing Mayo scissors, sharp dissection of the cyst from its bed was performed. The cyst was mobilized further with the handle of the scalpel. The rectal wall was easily distinguished from the cyst by inserting a finger into the rectum during the dissection. This was performed utilizing a double-gloved hand. Following removal of the Bartholin's gland cyst, the vestibular bulb beneath the Bartholin's duct was located and the entire cavity was obliterated by approximating the walls with fine delayed absorbable suture material after excision of the cyst.

Hemostasis was judged to be excellent and the operative site was thoroughly irrigated with Betadine solution. Approximation of the vaginal mucosa was accomplished with a continuous mucosal suture of 1–0 _____ (delayed absorbable) material. The patient tolerated the procedure well and hemostasis was judged to be excellent. The patient went to the Recovery Room in a stable condition.

---

### Important points/pearls

- Broad-spectrum antibiotics are usually helpful during treatment of Bartholin's gland abscesses since they contain mixed bacterial organisms.
- Excision is usually a last resort after Word catheter placement or marsupialization has been tried, since complications include hemorrhage, painful scar formation, hematoma, and cellulitis.
- Indications for excision include persistent or recurrent abscesses or cysts. Malignancies need to be ruled out in postmenopausal women.

# Burch retropubic suspension (Cooper's ligament modification of MMK)

**Technique**

After the intra-abdominal procedure was completed and peritoneum closed, the dissection into the space of Retzius was started using blunt dissection and only sharp dissection into areas of distortion and/or obliteration. Bleeding was controlled with pressure, careful fulguration, and individual ligature, as was necessary.

The dissection was carried down toward the inferior aspect of the symphysis to within 1 cm of the external urethral meatus. With the patient in the semi-frog position and a #24 Foley catheter in the bladder, two fingers were placed into the vagina and the anterior vagina was elevated so that proper and accurate placement of sutures could be performed. Using the catheter as a urethral guide and the balloon as a spot for the trigonal and bladder neck area, sutures of #1 delayed absorbable material were placed. These sutures were placed in the paraurethral tissues of the endopelvic fascia and bladder neck and then placed into the iliopectineal ligament (Cooper's ligament), avoiding any trauma to the periosteum. Two throws were placed on each side of the vaginal wall and urethra. Gloves and gown were then changed and the sutures were then tied and cut in pairs from below upward. At no time did it appear that any needle was placed into the urethra or bladder wall.

**Important points (prior to closing)**

- Suprapubic Silastic tube (#12F) can be inserted through the skin and into the bladder under direct vision for abdominal drainage prior to closure of the incision. A small Penrose drain is placed on either side of the midline in the operative area if there is residual venous bleeding, and the wound is closed per routine.
- If there is any uncertainty about proper location of the suture along the bladder neck, the surgeon should not hesitate to open the dome of the bladder transversely in order to place the suture under direct vision. Improper placement of the needle will probably cause symptoms of recurrent frequency and urgency.
- This procedure and the MMK are often the abdominal approaches to treatment of GSI as opposed to vaginal procedures such as the

Pereyra and Stamey techniques. This procedure can also be performed laparoscopically (see laparoscopic section of this book). The sling procedures, including IVS, TVTs, TOPs, and others, have replaced many of the previous 'gold standard' procedures such as the MMK for urinary incontinence.

- An enterocele develops in 8% of these cases post-op due to change in the pelvic axis. The Burch is a poorly suited procedure for a patient with a small vaginal size or poor vaginal mobility.
- Remember that 80–85% of patients will have improved outcome no matter which technique is used (with the exception of the sling that is >90% effective) and that surgical failures often result from poor preoperative evaluation of the etiology of GSI.

# Cesarean section

**An overview**

There are three main methods of transcribing a C-section that will be mentioned in this book:

(1) the Kerr (low transverse uterine) incision, which is the most common
(2) the Krönig (low vertical uterine) incision
(3) the C-section for breech extraction.

The Krönig incision can also be extended into a classical incision that becomes very useful in emergency situations such as anterior placenta previa, preterm fetuses, or abnormal lies and/or compound presentations. Since the vertical incision still has indications but is rarely performed, it is only mentioned here. The C-section for breech, however, still makes up 10% of C-section indications (according to National Center for Health Statistics National Hospital Discharge Surveys). Therefore, a sample transcription of both a Kerr C-section and C-section for breech extraction will be given.

Variations in technique to enter the uterus should be kept in mind. One may need to utilize Allis clamps to lift the small uterine incision away from the infant as the incision is carried deeper into the uterus. This can be extremely important with an occipital posterior position, where a facial laceration or orbital injury could occur. Scissors or manual extension of the incision can be performed and even using the Poly CS-57 uterine absorbable stable device might be preferred. (At present, information is limited on long-term follow-up on patients and experience in VBAC when the stapling device was used.) If this type of device is to be used, however, it is just as important (or possibly more important) to insert a finger into the uterus to clear fetal tissue from the area to be stapled. The finger is then placed protectively between the stapler and the fetus to avoid entrapment of fetal tissue during introduction of the device. No matter what method is used to enter the uterus, it is most important to aim the extensions of the incision toward the fundus in order to avoid the major uterine vessels.

Infection and endometritis are the two most significant complications of the C-section procedure. For the purpose of this book, there are a few suggestions that might be recommended to include in transcription of the procedure. One should describe the appearance and odor of the amniotic fluid upon entry into the uterus. It is almost considered the standard of care to administer an antibiotic after cord clamping except in very low-risk patients. Some physicians prefer to give an antibiotic in regards to all C-sections. There have been some sources of literature that propose lavage as an excellent prophylactic antibiotic (usually an example might be 2 g of Mandol mixed with 1–2 liters of normal saline). However, it appears that the less cumbersome intravenous method has become the standard of care for the prophylaxis of C-section in labor. It is important to mention the type and amount of antibiotic used during surgery. There are many other methods that might help reduce the infection rate in each C-section. The removal of the outer doubled glove after it has been adjacent to the vagina during the delivery of the infant is one suggestion. Removal of the scalp electrode before or during the procedure (if there is one present) is another. One may also try to decrease the number of vaginal exams prior to the procedure if possible. Some of these are certainly just suggestions and have not been proven as an acceptable standard of care.

Removing the infant can be accomplished by the surgeon's hand, with the aid of a uterine head elevator, or with a suction device (Mityvac, CMI, or any soft silicone vacuum extractor cup). If a suction device is used, the amount of pressure applied to the infant's scalp should be recorded. This amount should not exceed the following:

(1) 580 mmHg
(2) 21 inches Hg
(3) 10 lb/in$^2$
(4) 0.7 kg/cm$^2$.

One might instead record that the VE pressures have remained in the green zone of 35–45 cmH$_2$O or 350–450 mmHg. These are the same recommendations for vaginal vacuum extractions. The placement is also the same. The center of the cup should be placed over the sagittal suture, 3 cm in front of the posterior fontanelle, and no maternal tissue should be trapped along the edge and underneath the cup. Pulls should be coordinated with the assistant's fundal pressure during C-section just as pulls are coordinated with maternal pushing efforts during vaginal extraction.

Infant statistics are often mentioned during the procedure or in the pre-procedure format. It is important to record the findings at the time of surgery so that this information can be easily retrieved if needed at a later time. This is usually transcribed as follows:

Infant statistics:

(1) sex
(2) Apgar score
(3) weight
(4) umbilical cord analysis: ABG _____ VBG _____

After the delivery of the infant and hemostasis is obtained, comment in regards to the appearance of the remainder of the viscera is important. A standard part of any C-section is examination of adnexa, including ovaries, fallopian tubes, and related structures. Removal, to avoid probable torsion, is usually reserved for larger hydatoids. In general, because leiomyomas are vascular and likely to regress, one should not attempt to remove one at C-section unless it has an easily accessible and/or avascular pedicle.

The abdomen should be checked while the patient's incision allows for adequate exposure. If the appendix contains a fecalith or appears abnormal, one should not hesitate to remove it. It can be embarrassing if the patient has acute appendicitis within a few hours after completion of surgery. The author has had this experience. One should transcribe all of these important points. The following pages give some sample transcriptions of Cesarean section dictations.

---

**Important points/pearls**

- Types of incision into uterus
  Kerr (low transverse):   most common
  Krönig (low vertical):   rare, but indicated in unusual circumstances (backdown transverse lies, etc.)
  Breech extraction:   using either of above

- Variations of entry into uterus
  Use of Allis clamps if necessary to lift myometrium away from infant and increase exposure.
  Extension of uterine incision
      scissors
      manual
      poly CS–57 absorbable staple device
  Important points:
      - avoid injury to fetus below incision!
      - aim incision upward to avoid major vessels bilaterally.

- infection/endometriosis
      Describe appearance and odor of amniotic fluid.
      Antibiotic after clamping cord.
      Lavage or intravenously?
      Consider double gloving and removing outer glove that was in lower uterine segment.
      Decrease number of vaginal exams prior to surgery.

- Record method of delivery
      Hand
      Uterine head elevator
      Suction device (Mityvac, CMI, etc.)
          Record pressure applied
              Pressure not to exceed:
              (1)   580 mmHg
              (2)   21 inches Hg
              (3)   10 lb/in$^2$
              (4)   0.7 kg/cm$^2$

---

- Record infant statistics
  Sex, Apgars, weight, and umbilical cord analysis (ABG, VBG, etc.)
- Note:
  Hemodynamics
  Appearance of viscera
  Exam of adnexa
  Removal of any large hydatoids to avoid torsion but mention of any leiomyoma unless on an easily accessible or avascular pedicle
  Appearance and/or removal of appendix
  Closure

## CESAREAN SECTION FOR BREECH EXTRACTION

### Technique

Patient was prepped and draped in the usual manner for a low Pfannenstiel abdominal incision. The incision was carried down through the subcutaneous tissue to the fascia. The fascia was incised with the scalpel blade and extended in a smiling fashion by sharp dissection using the Mayo scissors. The underlying muscle tissue was sharply dissected away from overlying fascia. The peritoneum was entered with sharp dissection using the Metzenbaum scissors and two hemostats to lift the entry site away from underlying abdominal viscera. The bladder was then sharply dissected away from the lower uterine segment using smooth forceps and Metzenbaum scissors. The bladder flap retractor was then placed between the uterus and bladder to expose the lower uterine segment. Incision was carried out using the scalpel and consideration was made as to whether to perform a vertical uterine incision or a low uterine incision because of the abnormal presentation. It was felt that, since the infant was not estimated to be extremely large, a low cervical incision should be attempted with the idea that a possible T-incision be made if necessary.

An incision was made in the uterus in a low transverse fashion and care was taken to expose the amniotic sac. The amniotic sac was then entered and the amniotic fluid encountered: this was clear. The extension of the low transverse incision was made with the surgeon's finger in a smiling fashion. The incision was opened to allow the surgeon's hand to be placed inside the uterine cavity. The surgeon's hand was placed into the intrauterine cavity and the fetal extremities were located. With mild fundal pressure the head was mildly pushed down and the feet extracted first. A towel was then wrapped around the legs and in a routine corkscrew fashion the sacrum was then delivered. Once the sacrum was delivered in a counterclockwise fashion, the body was delivered with very gentle pressure. Each shoulder was then delivered in a systematic fashion, and then, in a smiling bite Mauriceau maneuver, the fingers were placed into the oropharynx of the aftercoming head. The baby was gently removed from the intrauterine cavity with both mild fundal pressure and the Mauriceau maneuver. The oropharynx was thoroughly suctioned with the suction bulb and DeLee suction. The cord was then clamped and cut as the baby's oropharynx was continually suctioned. The outer glove of the right hand, which had been in the lower uterine segment, was removed and the baby's oropharynx was suctioned thoroughly with the suction bulb. The umbilical cord was clamped in sections for possible cord blood gas analysis and routine blood testing. The section closest to the infant was cut with scissors beyond the cord clamp and the infant was removed from the operative field by Dr _____ . The infant was spontaneously crying.

Pitocin (2 ampules) was given in the remaining _____ of Ringer's lactate already infiltrating. The patient was also given _____ (antibiotic). The placenta and remaining amniotic membrane were then manually removed from the intrauterine cavity. The intrauterine cavity was checked very carefully for any remaining products of conception and having made certain there was none, the uterine incision was reapproximated in two layers. The first layer was closed in an interlocking continuous 0 (delayed absorbable suture). The second layer was reapproximated over the first and the bladder was then reapproximated with 2-0 (delayed absorbable) continuous suture. After the uterus and adnexa were in the proper anatomical position in the pelvis, the abdomen was inspected and found to be normal in appearance (including the appendix). The peritoneum was closed with _____ in a continuous fashion. The fascia was reapproximated with 2-0 (delayed absorbable suture) in a continuous fashion. The subcutaneous tissue was then closed with 3-0 (absorbable) on a T-26 needle. The skin was then reapproximated with _____.

Bandage was applied. Sponge, lap, instrument, and needle counts were all correct. Estimated blood loss was _____. The patient was then moved to the Recovery Room in good condition.

---

**Author's notes**

Some obstetrical surgeons prefer to close the uterus in only one layer. Some do not reapproximate the bladder or peritoneum either. The above transcription involves closing the uterus in two layers, the bladder flap and peritoneum.

## KERR CESAREAN SECTION (LOW TRANSVERSE UTERINE INCISION)

### Technique

Patient was prepped and draped in the usual manner for a low Pfannenstiel abdominal incision. The incision was carried down through the subcutaneous tissue to the fascia. The fascia was incised with the scalpel blade and extended in a smiling fashion by sharp dissection using the Mayo scissors. The underlying muscle tissue was sharply dissected away from overlying fascia. The peritoneum was entered with sharp dissection using the Metzenbaum scissors and two hemostats to lift the entry site away from underlying abdominal viscera. The bladder was then sharply dissected away from the lower uterine segment using smooth forceps and Metzenbaum scissors. The bladder flap retractor was then placed between the uterus and bladder to expose the lower uterine segment.

Incision was carried out using the scalpel and entry into the uterus was made, being careful to expose the amniotic sac. Amniotic sac was entered and the fluid was noted to be clear and there was no foul odor. Extension of the incision into the uterus was carried out in a low transverse smiling fashion, being careful to avoid major vasculature along the lower uterine segment bilaterally.

The surgeon's hand was placed just inside the uterine cavity to gently lift the infant's head into view so as to expose the scalp in order to place the Mityvac suction cup. —— mmHg was applied in order to bring the head out of the uterus. The outer glove of the right hand that had been in the lower uterine segment was removed and the baby's oropharynx was suctioned thoroughly with the suction bulb. The remainder of the infant was then delivered and the umbilical cord was clamped in sections for cord blood gas analysis and routine blood testing. The section closest to the infant was cut with scissors beyond the cord clamp and the infant was removed from the operative field by Dr _____. The infant was crying spontaneously.

Pitocin (2 ampules) was given in the remaining _____ ml of Ringer's lactate already infiltrating. The patient was also given _____ (antibiotic). The placenta and remaining amniotic membrane were then manually removed from the intrauterine cavity. The intrauterine cavity was checked very carefully for any remaining products of conception and, having made certain there was none, the uterine incision was reapproximated in two layers.

The first layer was closed in an interlocking continuous 0-delayed absorbable suture. The second layer was reapproximated over the first layer using a continuous Lembert-style 0-delayed absorbable suture. Hemostasis was excellent and the bladder was then reapproximated with 2-0 delayed absorbable continuous suture. After the uterus and adnexa were in the proper anatomical position in the pelvis, the abdomen was inspected and found to be normal in appearance (including the appendix). The peritoneum was closed with _____ in a continuous fashion. The fascia was reapproximated with _____ (2-0 delayed absorbable) suture in a continuous fashion. The subcutaneous tissue was then closed with _____ 3-0 (absorbable) on a _____ needle. The skin was then reapproximated with _____ . Bandage was applied. Sponge, lap, instrument, and needle counts were all correct. Estimated blood loss was _____ . The patient then was moved to the Recovery Room in good condition.

---

**Author's notes**

This C-section sample suggested using a Mityvac extraction device. The surgeon's hand is probably the most common method of lifting the head out of the uterus. However, the vacuum extractor is usually the author's preference because of the seemingly smaller uterine incision that is necessary, thus decreasing blood loss.

Some sources have suggested placing moist laparotomy cloths in the pericolic gutters prior to making the uterine incision to absorb amniotic fluid, blood, and meconium, in an attempt to decrease postoperative ileus.

# Cerclage

**Important points/pearls**

- Contraindications to most cerclages include:

    (1) uterine bleeding
    (2) uterine contractions
    (3) chorioamnionitis
    (4) cervical dilatation >4 cm
    (5) polychorioamnionitis
    (6) known fetal anomaly
    (7) ruptured membranes.

    Exceptions to the above can include emergency cerclage procedures during advanced preterm labor, bulging membranes, or when labor has been arrested prior to such cerclages (see Wurm or Saskatchewan procedures) – especially in rural settings when transfer of the patient to a tertiary nursery may be of utmost importance.
- Anesthesia is most often spinal or epidural.
- Make deep enough bites to reinforce but not so deep to rupture the membranes or injure the bladder.
- During the Shirodkar cerclage, many physicians have started tying their knots posteriorly to avoid erosion into the bladder. However, during McDonald's cerclage, leave the knot in the anterior position to facilitate removal. The McDonald's cerclage is the most common. The author performs a double cerclage (using two sutures and two knots) to strengthen and improve the results.
- Abdominal cerclage should be performed only when vaginal cerclage has failed or is not feasible (secondary to the higher complication rate and need for two abdominal procedures).
- Pre-op evaluation:

    (1) delay timing of cerclage until about 14–26 weeks (preferably 14 weeks) EGA (estimated gestation age)
    (2) ultrasound (to rule out major anomalies and confirm viability)
    (3) screen for gonorrhea (GC), chlamydia, and group B beta streptococcus (GBBS) via cultures and treat if necessary
    (4) no coitus for at least 1 week prior and 1 week after cerclage.

## TRANSABDOMINAL CERVICAL CERCLAGE

### Technique

The peritoneal reflection was transversely divided and the bladder advanced away from the lower uterine segment using both blunt and sharp dissection.

The space between the ascending and descending branches of the uterine arteries lateral to the cervicouterine junction was identified. The area was developed carefully by blunt dissection medially to the uterine arteries and veins and laterally to the connective tissue of the uterine isthmus using long right-angle forceps with tapered jaws. The assistant provided upward traction on the uterine fundus so as to expose the internal os and tense the vessels.

After a 1–2 cm tunnel had been developed in the avascular space, the broad ligament's posterior leaf was punctured with right-angle forceps. A 15 cm segment of 0.5 cm Mersilene tape was passed through the aperture under direct vision so as to prevent slippage of the forceps or inclusion of tissue with ribbon and consequent laceration of thin-walled veins. The same was performed on the contralateral side.

The Mersilene band was passed around the uterine isthmus and over the posterior peritoneum at the level of the uterosacral ligament insertions. The band was flat, snug, and compressed the intervening tissue. The band was secured anteriorly with a single square knot and the cut ends were fixed to the band with _____ (2 or 3-0 fine silk or non-absorbable) sutures.

(Closure of peritoneum and abdomen is now transcribed.)

---

### Author's notes

Pfannenstiel incision is recommended for 12–15 weeks' gestation but a vertical incision is advised thereafter. Transcribe the incision and entry into the peritoneum.

The transabdominal cerclage is used for:

(1) traumatic cervix
(2) congenital shortening of the cervix
(3) previous failed vaginal cerclage
(4) advanced cervical effacement.

## CONE CERCLAGE

### Technique

Routine prep and drape was carried out with the patient under general anesthesia. A _____ (#16 Foley) catheter was inserted into the bladder. The cervix was visualized after weighted speculum and _____ (Sims) retractor was placed into the vagina. A single-tooth tenaculum was placed on the anterior lip of the cervix close to the bladder reflection and one on the posterior lip.

The entire ectocervix was injected with vasopressin (20 units in 60 ml normal saline) until the cervix blanched. Lateral hemostatic sutures were placed at the 10 o'clock and 2 o'clock positions on the cervix using _____ (2-0 polyglycolic acid) sutures.

A standard McDonald's cerclage (may transcribe complete procedure here) using _____ (#1 nylon or 5 Ethibond) suture was then inserted as high and as close to the internal cervical os as technically possible without reflection of the bladder.

The cervical cone was cut using a _____ (#11 surgical blade) with a marker suture placed at the 12 o'clock position on the specimen. Following excision of the cone, the McDonald's suture was tied with the knot placed anteriorly. A _____ (2 inch iodoform) packing was placed in the vagina and instrumentation removed from the vagina. The patient went to the Recovery Room and fetal viability was confirmed.

### Author's notes

Cone cerclage in pregnancy was described in *Am J Obstet Gynecol* **77**(2) February 1991. All patients are pregnant whose cytology or pathology is suggestive of invasive or microinvasive carcinoma, unsatisfactory colposcopy, or lesions in the endocervical canal for which the upper limits of the lesion cannot be visualized and endocervical curettage cannot be done.

### Emergency procedures of cerclage

Usually, elevation of the bulging membranes needs to be performed prior to these cerclages:

(1) overfill bladder with 1000 ml saline
(2) Trendelenburg (with or without Foley displacement)
(3) use sponge stick with condom cover.

## EMERGENCY PROCEDURE: SASKATCHEWAN PROCEDURE

### Technique

After _____ (general or epidural) anesthesia, the patient was placed in steep Trendelenburg position. Routine prep and drape was performed along with vaginal irrigation with _____ (cefamandole) solution. Weighted speculum and necessary _____ (Sims) retractors were placed to expose the cervix.

Eight cervical stay sutures of _____ (#0 silk or Mersilene) were attached to the edges of the effaced cervix with a free needle. Care was taken to avoid the cervical edges with instruments and retractors so as to avoid perforation of the membranes.

Traction on the stay sutures was carried out to move the protruding membranes back into the uterine cavity.

Once the membranes are displaced upward, two rows of #1 _____ (silk or stout Mersilene) suture are placed as high as possible into the substance of the effaced cervix. These sutures are tightened and tied anteriorly. Half of the stay sutures are removed and the others are tied across the external os to close the cervix effectively. Vaginal instrumentation was removed and the patient taken to the Recovery Room in Trendelenburg position. She was given terbutaline sulfate 0.25 mg subcutaneously to ensure uterine relaxation. Fetal viability was confirmed in the Recovery Room.

### Author's notes

Traction on the stay sutures is carried out to move the protruding membranes back into the uterine cavity. If the membranes are not completely prolapsed, a deflated 30 ml Foley balloon catheter can be inserted into the external os of the cervix and the balloon filled with water to displace the forewaters above the level of the internal os. Once the cerclage is placed, deflate the balloon and remove the catheter. If all fails to reduce the bulging bag, insert an amniocentesis needle *suprapubically* or under ultrasonic guidance to withdraw several hundred ml of fluid to deflate the bulge.

## EMERGENCY PROCEDURE: WURM PROCEDURE

### Techniques

After deep general anesthesia was obtained and steep Trendelenburg position was achieved, the vulva was prepped with _____ (Betadine,

Hibiclens) solution. The vagina was irrigated with _____ (Mandol or an antiseptic) solution. The membranes were gently pushed back into the uterine cavity with a sponge holding forceps (covered with a condom if available).

The assistant gently held the bulging membranes back as double mattress sutures of _____ (5 Ethibond) were placed from 2 o'clock to 10 o'clock positions and back in at 8 o'clock to 4 o'clock positions to be tied at 3 o'clock position. The next suture was placed at 1 o'clock to 5 o'clock and back in at 7 o'clock to 11 o'clock position and was tied at the 12 o'clock position.

Vaginal instrumentation was removed, the patient kept in Trendelenburg position, and fetal viability was confirmed in the Recovery Room. The patient was also given _____ (prophylactic antibiotic).

## LASER CONE CERCLAGE

### Technique

After the epidural anesthesia was found to be adequate, routine prep with _____ solution and drape was completed. The laser bivalve speculum was connected to the smoke evacuation and blood evacuation system. The laser incision was outlined by short bursts of laser energy, leaving a margin of 2–3 mm of normal cervical tissue. A power setting of 30 watts was utilized in continuous energy, with a spot size of 0.5 mm. The power setting was increased to 40 watts while lasering into the deeper areas of the cervical stroma. The cervix was blotted with an acetic acid solution during the entire procedure. The laser incisions were deepened to at least 3–5 mm straight into the cervical stroma, so that the cone could be easily grasped with several different pairs of laser Iris hooks to enable the beam to be angled toward the endocervical canal.

The conization was without complications and the cone easily shelled out so that the apex of the cone was able to be severed with a short burst of 40 watts of laser energy. (Some prefer to use a scalpel to sever the apex.) Following the removal of the cone, the 12 o'clock position was tagged with a safety pin. The cone was sent to pathology. The laser crater was then swabbed thoroughly with 4% acetic acid solution and bleeding points were lasered with 30 and 40 watts of power with a defocused beam and then swabbed again with 4% acetic acid solution. The entire crater was then soaked with Monsel's solution on a cotton swab and held against the crater for approximately 45 seconds.

Hemostasis was _____ (excellent, good, or describe blood control or loss – the following cerclage portion of the procedure usually also aids in control of any remaining oozing or blood loss).

Utilizing a _____ (#5 Ethibond suture or 5 mm Mersilene), this was inserted in the 11 o'clock position and brought out at the 10 o'clock position. The suture was then brought around the 9 o'clock position and placed in around the 8 o'clock position. It was then brought out about the 7 o' clock position, brought around the cervix, and replaced at about the 5 o'clock position. The suture was then brought out around the 3 o'clock position and replaced in the 2 o'clock position, bringing the suture back out at around the 1 o'clock position to tie with the original suture, which was still in the 11 o'clock position. This was tied at the 12 o'clock position until the cervix demonstrated closure utilizing the finger.

---

**Author's notes**

Cone cerclage in pregnancy was described in *Am J Obstet Gynecol* **77**(2) February 1991, and has been successfully adapted to 'laser' cone cerclage by the author, having what he believes to be much less blood loss. All patients that are pregnant, whose cytology or pathology is suggestive of invasive or microinvasive carcinoma, unsatisfactory colposcopy, or lesions in the endocervical canal for which the upper limits of the lesion cannot be visualized and endocervical curettage cannot be done, are candidates for cone cerclage.

## McDONALD'S CERCLAGE

**Technique**

The patient was prepped and draped in the usual manner for a vaginal approach. A weighted speculum was placed into the vagina and, utilizing a right-angle retractor in the vagina, the cervix was located and grasped with an Allis clamp.

Utilizing a _____ (#5 Ethibond suture or 5 mm Mersilene band), this was inserted in the 11 o'clock position and brought out at the 10 o'clock position. The suture is then brought around the 9 o'clock position and placed in around the 8 o'clock position and brought out about the 7 o'clock position. It is then brought around the cervix and replaced at about the 5 o'clock position and brought out around the 3 o'clock position and replaced in the 2 o'clock position. Bringing the suture back out at around the 1 o'clock position, it is then tied with the original suture, which was still in the 11 o'clock position. This was tied at the 12 o'clock position until the cervix demonstrated closure, utilizing the finger. (*This process can be repeated for additional strength.*)

This entire purse-string suture was started anteriorly as high as possible and above the area where the smooth adherent mucosa covering the cervix joins the more mobile rugose vaginal mucosa. The suture was placed deeply, especially in the posterior portion, since it is this area that most often subsequently pulls out. The patient was instructed prior to anesthesia that she must remain at bedrest for a minimum of a week following the cerclage and she was also given sedation and prophylactic antibiotics. All instruments were removed from the vagina and the patient went to the Recovery Room in good condition.

## SHIRODKAR CERCLAGE

### Technique

After routine prep and drape, a weighted speculum and _____ (Sims) retractor were placed into the vagina to expose the cervix.

The vaginal mucosa was incised transversely at the anterior and posterior cervical vaginal junction after injecting approximately _____ (20 ml) of 1:1000 solution of epinephrine along the anterior vaginal fornix and posteriorly at the level of the uterosacral ligaments. The incisions are extended laterally about 1.5 cm on either side. The areolar tissue was separated bluntly by spreading _____ (Metzenbaum) scissors until the vesicouterine fascia was identified. The bladder was then advanced a short distance and then retracted. The posterior vaginal wall was similarly incised but care was taken not to enter the peritoneum.

Allis clamps were then used to compress the lateral paracervical tissue containing the blood supply. The anterior and posterior edges of the cut vaginal mucosa were then grasped and a 5 mm Mersilene tape swagged to double-armed tapered needles was passed between the blood vessels laterally and the fibromuscular substance of the cervix. The suture was tightened as firmly as possible while remaining flat and avoiding perforation of the cervix or membranes.

Another high _____ (2-0 silk) suture was placed through the cervical fascia to secure the tape and prevent sliding of the cerclage downward. The anterior and posterior vaginal incisions were closed with interrupted 0- _____ (chromic or polyglycolic acid) sutures.

---

### Author's notes

The Shirodkar is more difficult to perform and is used with previous McDonald failures. It involves submucosal placement and more closely approaches the level of the internal os.

---

# Conization of cervix

---

**Important points/pearls**

Indications of excisional conization (pre-op):

(1) no lesion is visible colposcopically (or lesion disappears into the canal)
(2) entire transformation zone is not visible
(3) cytology abnormality not consistent with tissue diagnosis
(4) endocervical curettage (ECC) indicative of disease in the canal
(5) intraepithelial lesion or microinvasive cancer is present in ECC or direct biopsy
(6) cytologic or biopsy evidence of premalignant or malignant *glandular* epithelium is detected.

LEEP conization is not included, as this is most often an office procedure and not transcribed. (See LEEP for this type of procedure.)

- Specimens should be excised in a single piece whether performed with scalpel or laser.
- Twelve o'clock position is identified with suture or safety pin.
- If it is uncertain whether all pathology has been removed with the cone specimen, curette the upper margins of the uterine canal to rule out pathology above the upper margin of the cone.

## COLD KNIFE CONIZATION

**Technique**

After the patient arrived in the Operating Room, preoperative vaginal examination was deferred and the routine intravaginal prep was not performed. The cervix was exposed with the patient in the lithotomy position and buttocks extended over the edge of the table. This was performed with a weighted _____ (Auvard or New York) speculum and a vaginal retractor. Lugol's stain was placed into the vagina and bilateral holding sutures were placed into the cervix laterally at 3 o'clock and 9 o'clock positions beyond the margins of the Schiller light epithelium. With traction on the cervix, the cervical stroma was infiltrated with approximately 50 ml of 1:200 000 solution of Neo-Synephrine in a circumferential manner. The cervix was seen to blanch and increase somewhat in size. An identifying suture was placed at the 12 o'clock position on the specimen with a single suture placed in the cervical stroma.

The uterine canal was then sounded gently and the sound was left in place to mark the course of the endocervical canal. A circular incision was then made outside the identifying suture and the Schiller light margin, beginning posteriorly with the tip of the blade directed against the metal probe in the cervical canal. The specimen was then fully excised and the tissue was given to the scrub nurse and was sent in this condition to Pathology, being careful not to place the tissue in fixative at this time.

Sturmdorf sutures were then placed in the posterior lip first, utilizing a #1 _____ (delayed absorbable) suture on a large cutting needle. The suture was placed so as to pick up the posterior flap of the mucosa in the midline near the edge. The suture was directed high into the endo-cervical canal, passing through the wall of the cervical canal out through the portio of the posterior cervical lip near the fornia approximately 2 cm from the site of the initial suture. As the mucosal flap was pulled forward, the other end of the suture was threaded into the cutting needle and the process of suturing through the cervical canal was repeated. The two ends of the suture emerged on the posterior surface of the cervix approximately 0.5 cm apart. Firm traction on this suture pulled the posterior mucosal flap well into the newly made cervical canal and the suture was tied; the procedure was repeated on the anterior lip.

Superficial electrocoagulation of the bleeding points in the cervical stroma was performed, followed by application of gelfoam sponge to necessary cervical defects. This was held in place with a vaginal pack that will be removed in approximately 24 hours. Hemostasis was judged to be excellent during the entire procedure.

## LASER CONIZATION OF CERVIX

### Technique

The patient was placed on the Operating Room table in the lithotomy position and, following careful pelvic exam, the laser speculum was placed into the vagina and the cervix was swabbed thoroughly with 4% acetic acid solution. The paracervical anesthetic was placed at the 8 o'clock, 4 o'clock, and 12 o'clock positions and the laser bivalve speculum was connected to the smoke evacuation and blood evacuating system. The laser incision was outlined by short bursts of laser energy, leaving a margin of 2–3 mm of normal cervical tissue. A power setting of 30 watts was utilized in continuous energy, with a spot size of 0.5 mm.

The power setting was increased to 40 watts while lasering into the deeper areas of the cervical stroma. The cervix was blotted with an acetic acid solution during the entire procedure. The laser incisions were deepened to at least 3–5 mm straight into the cervical stroma so that the cone could be easily grasped with several different pairs of laser Iris hooks and thus enable the beam to be angled toward the endocervical canal.

The conization was without complications and the cone easily shelled out so that the apex of the cone was able to be severed with a short burst of 40 watts of laser energy. (Some prefer to use a scalpel to sever the apex.) Following the removal of the cone, the 12 o'clock position was tagged with a safety pin. The cone was sent to Pathology. The laser crater was then swabbed thoroughly with 4% acetic acid solution and bleeding points were lasered with 30 and 40 watts of power with a defocused beam and then swabbed again with 4% acetic acid solution. The entire crater was then soaked with Monsel's solution on a cotton swab and held against the crater for approximately 45 seconds. Hemostasis was excellent. Q-tips were also used to bring about excellent hemostasis.

The patient has been given routine outpatient laser instructions and will be seen in approximately 12 weeks for follow-up cytology and possible colposcopy.

# Cystoscopy

**Important points/pearls**

It is most important for every surgical gynecologist to have experience and privileges in performing cystoscopy:

(1) In the office, cystoscopy allows one to be able to assess ISD (intrinsic sphincter deficiency) without complicated urodynamic machines.

(2) Cystoscopy also allows one to be able to assess and rule out the bladder as the etiology of chronic pelvic pain such as IC (interstitial cystitis). If one is uncertain about Huhner's ulcers or other pathological findings, one can perform the intravesical potassium sensitivity test (through a #10F pediatric tube instill 40 ml of 0.4 (mmol/liter) KCl of $H_2O$ or saline into the bladder). Intravesical treatments such as 4–6 mg/kg of 5% lidocaine and equal volume 8.4% $NaHCO_3$, Elmiron 100 mg t.i.d. or 10 000–20 000 units of heparin in 20 ml 1% lidocaine and 3 ml 8.4% $NaHCO_3$ and many other multimodal therapies can be used to treat this condition if discovered.

(3) In the Surgical Suite, one can check the ureteral orifices for bilateral spillage of indigo carmine, if one suspects possible ureteral injury after a difficult pelvic case.

(4) During and after sling procedures, the placement of slings and/or sutures *must* be continually checked and rechecked to avoid missing an inadvertent injury to the bladder wall. A 70° cystoscope is best for evaluating as much of the inside of the bladder as possible.

(5) During periurethral bulking procedures, it is best to use a 0° urethroscope so that the urethrovesical junction can be best evaluated during injections.

## Technique

*Since the cystoscopy is usually performed along with another procedure, the transcription will begin as follows:*

The cystoscope was attached to camera lens and all tubing. The cystoscope was then gently advanced as required to observe the urethra, UV junction, and bladder wall. The entire bladder was further filled with _____ (250–300 ml) of normal saline and both ureteral orifices were visualized. *Transcribe whether both orifices spilled dye at this point if noted.* The entire bladder (including anterior, posterior, lateral walls, including the trigone) were noted to be normal without injury, suture, or bruising. At this point, the cystoscope was removed while observing the entire movement throughout the procedure. The bladder was then emptied per catheter.

# Dilatation and curettage

---

**Important points/pearls**

- Endocervical curettage (ECC) is usually performed with a Kevorkian curette up to the internal os, usually at least twice around with short, firm strokes, without catching portions of external os.
- Sound the uterus *only after* ECC to avoid pushing tissue from the cervix into the uterus.
- Try to predict severe retroversion or antiversion so as to avoid easy perforation.
- Remember to note whether or not abnormal tissue was present.

Points regarding elective and/or therapeutic abortions can be seen under *Suction Dilatation and Evacuation (D & E)*, since this is the most common method of evacuation of POC (products of conception) rather than dilatation and curettage (D & C).

## Technique

The patient was placed on the operating table in the lithotomy position. Careful pelvic examination was performed to locate the position of the uterine corpus. The vagina and the perineum were cleaned with _____ in the routine fashion.

The cervix was grasped with tenaculum and gently drawn toward the vaginal outlet. A small curette was utilized to obtain endocervical curettings. These were obtained on Telfa pad and handed off to be sent to Pathology. A sound was then passed through the cervical canal into the uterine cavity. This was done carefully to avoid creating a false passage. The length of the uterine cavity was _____ cm. Once the position of the uterus, the length of the uterine cavity, and angulation between the cervical canal and uterine cavity had been ascertained, the sound was removed and the cervical canal was dilated with a small dilator. After a 3 mm dilator was passed, successively larger ones were used. After dilatation of 9 mm was reached, the dilatation was discontinued.

A gauze was placed into the posterior vaginal fornix along with posterior weighted speculum retractor with a Telfa pad on top of the sponge so that blood and endometrium removed from the uterus would fall onto it. The uterine cavity was explored initially in search of any endometrial polyps with the polyp forceps. The forceps were moved systematically across the dome of the uterus and the anterior and posterior walls. The procedure was repeated several times and then the curettage was performed with a sharp curette. This was performed in a systematic manner in which the area of the endometrial cavity was covered. The procedure utilizing the polyp forceps was again repeated several times after the uterine wall had been curetted to make certain that there was no area of endometrial cavity that polyp or pathology might have been missed. A malleable, bluntly serrated curette was then introduced again into the uterus and in a systematic manner the entire uterine cavity was curetted. Anterior, lateral, and posterior walls were scraped gently but firmly and finally the top of the cavity was scraped with a side-to-side movement. After appropriate endometrial curettings had been obtained, these were placed immediately in fixative, being careful not to mash or scrape the specimens. There was no fatty tissue or unusual tissue noted. Hemostasis was judged to be excellent and all instrumentation was removed from the vagina. The patient was removed to the Recovery Room in good condition.

# Exenteration

## ANTERIOR PELVIC EXENTERATION

Exploratory laparotomy, radical hysterectomy, radical cystectomy, bilateral salpingo-oophorectomy, periaortic and pelvic lymph node dissection, periaortic lymph adenectomy, bilateral, pelvic lymph adenectomy, bilateral, ileoconduit formation, and examination under anesthesia are included for completeness.

### Technique

After intermittent venous calf compression booties had been attached, a satisfactory level of general endotracheal anesthesia was induced and examination under anesthesia was carried out. A Foley catheter was inserted into the bladder and noted to return clear urine. The findings of examination under anesthesia are as dictated above. The patient was placed supine and prepped and draped in a sterile fashion. The abdomen was entered through a midline incision, extending up just to the left of the umbilicus. Exploration was carried out; all of the upper abdominal viscera were normal to palpation. There was no adenopathy appreciated. Exploration was carried out with the findings as noted above: i.e. a tumor in the vesicovaginal septum. The aortic nodes were negative for metastatic disease; therefore, it was felt advisable to proceed with anterior pelvic exenteration, which was accomplished as follows.

A self-retaining retractor had been placed and the bowels had been packed away superiorly. The pelvic spaces were opened by first dividing the round ligaments bilaterally with an LDS $CO_2$ power device. The peritoneum overlying the bladder was incised high to the anterior parietal peritoneum and then the peritoneum in this area was dissected down and freed off of the bladder surface so the peritoneum could be used for reconstruction of the pelvic floor later. The actual muscularis of the dome of the bladder was left to go with the surgical specimen to be extrapolated. The perivesical and perirectal spaces were developed bilaterally down to the level of the levator muscles of the pelvic floor. The rectovaginal system was opened and explored and found to be free of tumor. The posterior vagina looked as though it had not been encroached upon; therefore, it was elected to proceed with anterior exenteration only. The rectovaginal septum was dissected down the length of the vagina and the colon pushed away posteriorly. An identical technique was used for management of the pelvic wall space and I will describe it in detail for the right side. Also described in detail below for the right side only is dissection of the ureter down to the area near the trigone. An identical operative technique was used on the contralateral side.

The right distal obliterated hypogastric artery was identified and the origin of the uterine artery from the more proximal internal iliac artery was identified. The soft tissues between the paravesical and pararectal spaces were mobilized. Dissection was then carried around anteriorly into the space of Retzius and the bladder was released from the infrapubic area. Blunt and sharp dissection was used to free up all the areolar tissue involved in the area of dissection. The course of the ureter was carefully identified and it was dissected down to the area where it coursed into the ureteric tunnel underneath the cardinal ligament. At this point the ureter was transected sharply with Potts scissors. The right pelvic side-wall was further dissected using clip-and-cut technique. The hypergastric artery was isolated and the anterior division was dissected free. The posterior division of the hypergastric artery was left in site. The anterior division was clamped and severed. Hemostasis on this artery was obtained by _____ (two ties of double 0 silk plus one metallic clip). Dissection was further carried down through the web, and the vein returning beneath the artery was carefully identified, dissected out, and ligated in a fashion similar to the artery above. Additional clips using a double side-wall clip and medial specimen single clip approach and cutting between them with the scissors was used to carry dissection all the way down to the levator muscles. The anterior lateral attachments of the bladder behind the symphysis were lysed with sharp dissection and bleeding was controlled with electrocautery. Dissection was carried down anteriorly to the level of the urethra.

Prior to all of this dissection, the infundibulopelvic ligaments bilaterally had been clamped, divided, and double ligated with _____ (0 Vicryl) sutures. The surgical specimen now consisted of uterus, tubes, ovaries, parametrium, paracolpium, vagina, and bladder. All of this was placed on the vertical upward traction and in the floor of the pelvis a sharp transverse incision went through the urethra and the lower third of the vagina, thus bringing the surgical specimen, which was handed off of the field. This was subsequently carried by the surgeon to the pathologist for proper orientation for permanent cuts.

The vagina was run with continuous _____ (0 chromic), incorporating some of the bleeding levator musculature. Additional hemostasis was obtained with electrocautery, as need be. The vaginal stump was then closed. The urethra was oversewn. The bleeders in the muscle bed were also oversewn and were electrocoagulated, as need be. The entire pelvic cavity defect was then copiously irrigated with saline solution. There was no continued bleeding.

As mentioned above, an aortic dissection had been accomplished prior to deciding to resect. That was done by simply resecting the ureters away from the aorta and vena cava and dissecting the precaval lymph nodes and the lymph nodes to the left of the lower abdominal aorta and submitting them for frozen section using a clip-and-cut technique.

Attention, at this time now, after resection of the anterior pelvis, was directed at dissection off of the common iliac lymph node chains bilaterally, the external iliac lymph node chains bilaterally, and the obturator lymph chains bilaterally. All of this was accomplished with sharp dissection using a clip-and-cut technique in the standard fashion. None of these nodes appeared to be involved with metastatic deposits, either at the time of dissection or at the prior time of palpation for anterior resection. Jackson–Pratt drains were placed in both sides of the pelvis and brought out through anterior abdominal stab wounds where they were fixed with _____ (1-0 silk) suture. An appropriate segment of ileum was then selected approximately _____ (8 cm) from the ileocecal valve and extending along for a segment length of approximately _____ (9 cm). Intraoperative pulse Doppler was used to confirm a satisfactory arterial arcade to this segment. GIAs were fired proximally and distally to the segment selected for ileoconduit formation. It is noted that, throughout the procedure, there was a good flow of urine noted through the cut ureters. An area for an ileal loop urostomy was selected in the right lower quadrant and a skin ellipse was removed. Dissection was carried down through the anterior abdominal wall. The distal end of the ileal loop was brought out through this, was opened with sharp dissections, and was formed into a rosebud formation using a triple-point fixation method using _____ (0 chromic) suture. The proposed conduit was then irrigated with Betadine. The proximal end of the conduit was intact. The ureters were then trimmed, cleaned, and splayed. The ureteral ileal anastomoses were then performed using _____ (4-0 GU chromic) on the splayed ureters on the ileal loop over stents. Retrograde injection of dilute Betadine solution showed that the anastomoses were watertight. Additional fatty tissue in the area was brought in to reinforce these anastomoses and the proximal end of the ileal loop was fixed down to the mesentery with several interrupted (0 chromic) sutures. Everything was then thoroughly irrigated in the abdomen and pelvis and the bowel were returned to as anatomical position as possible. The previously described peritoneal flap was used to help reperitonealize the floor of the pelvis. Sponge, instruments, and needles were removed and these counts were reported as correct times two. Intravenously injected indigo carmine followed by a bolus of fluid and Lasix was seen to have egress at the end of the urinary diversion. There was no leak at the anastomotic sites.

The anterior abdominal wall was closed with a modified Smead–Jones technique using figure-of-eight sutures of _____ (1-0 Prolene). The subcutaneous tissues were irrigated copiously with saline, Betadine, and saline and the skin edges were approximated with metallic clips. The sponge and instrument count was again reported as correct. The patient was transferred to the Recovery Room in satisfactory condition.

## Acknowledgment

This transcription was contributed by Dr Vernon Jobson, then reviewed and edited by Dr John E Turrentine.

## TOTAL PELVIC EXENTERATION

Examination under anesthesia; exploratory laparotomy; periaortic lymph node biopsies, including a low anterior colon resection with primary anastomosis and loop colostomy; and formation of ileourinary conduit and sigmoid colon neovagina are included in this transcription for completeness.

### Technique

The patient was brought to the Operating Room and intermittent venous calf compression boots were placed. Pulses were full and general anesthesia was induced. She was prepped in the usual manner for abdominal surgery and sterile draped. The abdomen was entered through a midline incision, carried in the midline just above the umbilicus. Exploration took place upon entering the abdomen. Please see author's notes. A self-retaining retractor was placed. Bowels were packed away superiorly. Attention was turned to the periaortic area and lymph nodes were sent for frozen section using a clip-and-cut technique. The frozen section returned benign.

Attention was turned anteriorly and the dissection carried down in the space of Retzius all the way to the level of the urethra. Pelvic side-wall space, specifically paravesical, perirectal spaces were joined with the dissection of the space of Retzius. Sequentially and bilaterally, the vascular structures were encountered and the paravesical and perirectal spaces were clamped, cut, and ligated with interrupted sutures all the way down to the pelvic floor. The distal ureters at this point were transected with Metzenbaum scissors and tagged with triple suture for later use. Additional dissection was carried down such that the specimen was fully mobilized from the six pelvic floor spaces, including the space of Retzius, space of Toldt, the paravesical spaces bilaterally, and the perirectal spaces bilaterally. Surgical specimen was placed on upward traction with the only two structures holding the specimen and the patient being the distal rectum and distal vaginal attachments. The vagina was then opened with sharp dissection and cut circumferentially. Circumferential running locking stitch was placed in the distal vaginal margin to control hemostasis. A small amount of dissection was then carried cephalad up the rectovaginal septum, thus leaving a small margin of distal rectum and the rectal sphincter intact. The rectum at this point was then transected and the operative specimen passed from the table.

Irrigation was performed in the pelvis. Hemostasis was achieved with electrocautery. When the space was judged to have good hemostasis, the pelvic floor was packed with hot, moist lap pads.

Attention was then turned to the more proximal colon, specifically the point of transection at the rectosigmoid. The descending colon was further mobilized up the splenic flexure, thus bringing the distal colon with adequate length down to the lower portions of the pelvis. It was judged at this point that the colon was adequate in length to create both a neovagina and primary anastomosis of the colon with loop colostomy.

First, the approximate _____ (12–15 cm) of distal rectosigmoid colon was transected by perforating the mesentery and crossclamping and dividing with the GIA stapling device. The mesentery was kept intact and this would later form the neovagina. The more proximal sigmoid colon was mobilized and brought down to the level of the distal rectal stump. The GIA staples were removed and primary anastomosis of the colon was performed using an end-to-end anastomosis. The mucosa was anastomosed using a running stitch circumferentially. Additional seromuscular sutures were placed circumferentially using interrupted simple silk sutures of _____ (000 silk). The anastomosis was palpated through the rectum and found to be intact, with adequate lumen and without leakage. The previously mentioned distal sigmoid colon segment was now brought to rest above the low anterior colon anastomosis at the level of the vagina. The GIA staples were removed and a primary anastomosis of the sigmoid colon to the vagina was made with first a running stitch of _____ (000 chromic) sewing mucosa to mucosa, followed by seromuscular sutures of approximating the bowel to distal vagina using _____ (000 silk). Again, palpation of both the rectum and the vagina showed that the rectal anastomosis was not compromised and had been further reinforced by this viable colon placed above the primary anastomosis. Mesenteric blood supply was judged to be intact on both structures. Irrigation was utilized in the operative field.

In the left midquadrant of the abdomen, skin incision was made circumferentially, thus creating the site for the loop colostomy. A loop of descending colon was brought through the stoma and the mesentery was perforated and a Hollister bridge was placed to stabilize this loop. It was further sutured to the skin with _____ (0 chromic) suture.

Some of the small bowel packs were removed and the distal ileum was visualized and a segment of distal ileum with a rainbow arterial arcade identified. Approximately _____ (12 cm segment) of ileum was selected and isolated at both ends with the GIA stapling device. In a converging, fan-shaped fashion, the pedicles were created in the ileomesentery so as to make a suitable immobile segment of ileum for construction of the urinary conduit. The distal and proximal ends of the resected ileum were then reanastomosed with a side-to-side, functional end-to-end GIA TA-35 anastomosis with staplers. The mesenteric defect was closed such that the conduit was placed below to reanastomose bowels. A circular incision was made in the right side of the abdomen and ileal stoma and was brought out through the stoma skin site. The ileal segment was found to be of adequate length. It was opened, the distal end with sharp dissection and a rosebud formation was created, thus securing the ileum to the skin. The conduit was then irrigated with _____ (a saline and Betadine mixture). The course of the distal ureters was identified. These were brought through the mesentery so that they could be attached to the ileal segment. Clamps were placed in a retrograde fashion through the ileostomy down the bowel and then sharp dissection was used to create small openings in the bowel such that the ureters could be anastomosed to the ileum. Anastomosis took place using multiple simple sutures of _____ (4-0 chromic) suture. Prior to closure of the ureteral ileal anastomotic sites, single J ureteral catheters were placed in a retrograde fashion up both ureters. The anastomotic site was oversewn and reinforced with an omental patch. Reflux of Betadine into the conduit showed the anastomosis was watertight. The base of the conduit was further secured with a few interrupted simple _____ (0 chromic) sutures to the pelvic side-wall and floor. Additional omentum was now brought in to further secure the conduit and fill the pelvis and pelvic floors as much as possible.

_____ (Jackson–Pratt) drains were placed in the pelvis and brought out through separate stab incisions in the lower abdomen and the cecum was further mobilized and brought down to the pelvis to further close the pelvic floor defect. Packs and retractors were removed. The small bowel was replaced in anatomical position as much as could be possibly done. Sponge, needle, and instrument counts were judged to be correct. The anterior abdominal wall was closed with multiple interrupted _____ (Prolene) sutures using _____ (Smead–Jones) closure technique. Subcutaneous tissue was irrigated with copious amounts of saline, followed by Betadine, followed by saline. Hemostasis was judged to be intact. The skin was approximated with skin clips. Dry dressing was placed on the wound. The urinary device was placed on the urinary stoma and clear urine was noted to be coming forth. A vaseline gauze was placed over the loop colostomy. The patient was considered to be stable throughout the entire procedure and was taken to the Recovery Room in stable condition. She was cared for in the intensive care unit postoperatively.

**Author's notes**

It is very important to transcribe indications and findings during dictation, but especially crucial in cases such as this – therefore, samples are included below.

## Sample

*Indications*

This patient has biopsy-proven recurrent squamous cell cancer of the cervix. She has been given preoperative external beam radiation therapy and now is brought to the Operating Room for definitive resection with curative intent.

**Findings** – At the time of surgery, opening of the paravesical and perirectal spaces to the pelvic floor failed to reveal any disease outside of the central recurrence. Periaortic lymph node biopsies were performed and frozen section was benign. The upper abdomen was totally negative, including right and left hemidiaphragm, right and left kidney, stomach, and small bowel. At the end of the procedure, the specimen was hand carried to Pathology and oriented for the pathologist, so that appropriate specimen orientation would assist us postoperatively and offer some prognostic indication.

## Acknowledgment

This transcription was contributed by Dr Charles H Pippitt, then reviewed and edited by Dr John E Turrentine.

# Fractional dilatation and curettage

## Technique

The patient was placed on the operating table in the lithotomy position. Careful pelvic examination was performed to locate the position of the uterine corpus. The vagina and the peritoneum were cleaned with _____ .

A weighted speculum was placed in the vagina. The cervix was grasped with tenaculum and gently drawn toward the vaginal outlet. A _____ (Gusberg, Kervorkian) curette was utilized to obtain endocervical curettings. These were obtained on a Telfa pad and passed to the circulating nurse to be sent to Pathology.

A sound was then passed through the cervical canal into the uterine cavity. This was done carefully to avoid creating a false passage. Once the position of the uterus, the length of the uterine cavity (describe length), and angulation between the cervical canal and uterine cavity had been ascertained, the sound was removed and the cervical canal was dilated with a small dilator. After a 3 mm dilator was passed, successively larger ones were used. After dilatation of (usually 9 mm) was reached, the dilatation was discontinued. Gauze was placed into the posterior vaginal fornix along with posterior weighted speculum retractor with a Telfa pad on top of the sponge so that blood and endometrium removed from the uterus would fall onto it.

The uterine cavity was explored initially in search of any endometrial polyps with the polyp forceps. The forceps were moved systematically across the dome of the uterus and the anterior and posterior walls. The procedure was repeated several times and then the curettage was performed with a sharp curette. This was performed in a systematic manner in which the entire area of the endometrial cavity was covered. The procedure utilizing the polyp forceps was again repeated several times after the uterine wall had been curetted to make certain that there was no area of endometrial cavity that polyp or pathology might have been missed. A malleable, bluntly serrated curette was then introduced again into the uterus and in a systematic manner the entire uterine cavity was curetted. Anterior, lateral, and posterior walls were scraped gently but firmly and finally the top of the cavity was scraped with a side-to-side movement. After appropriate endometrial curettings had been obtained, these were placed immediately in fixative, being careful not to mash or scrape the specimens. There was no fatty tissue or unusual tissue noted. Hemostasis was judged to be excellent and all instrumentation was removed from the vagina. Blood loss was minimal. The patient was removed to the Recovery Room in good condition.

# Groin and inguinal node dissection

**Technique**

The femoral canal was dissected in a manner that allowed the tissue to be removed from the surrounding artery and vein. Cloquet's nodes (nodes of Rosenmüller) were located at the femoral ring beneath the inguinal ligament. They were dissected with Metzenbaum scissors and sent for frozen section. (If these are negative for any metastatic disease, the dissection for vulvar disease can be considered complete.)

The deep inguinal chain was dissected by opening the inguinal canal from the external inguinal ring. The round ligament that passes into the canal from the peritoneal cavity (where the inguinal ring begins) was excised and the deep inguinal lymphatic tissue was removed.

The extraperitoneal pelvic lymphadenectomy was initiated by opening the external oblique muscle 2 cm above the inguinal ligament. The incision was extended as far laterally as necessary for exposure through the internal oblique and transversalis muscles. Retracting the peritoneum medially, the iliac vessels were exposed.

The external iliac, common iliac, and upper portion of hypogastric vessels were included in the dissection as the entire obturator space was thoroughly cleaned. The inferior epigastric artery and vein were ligated with 2-0 _____ (silk) suture. This was performed at the point where these vessels originated from the external iliac vessels, just inside the inguinal ligament, as they coursed upward to supply the abdominal wall. The ureter was displaced medially with the parietal peritoneum so as to avoid injury during the dissection.

Following dissection of necessary nodes, a _____ (Jackson–Pratt) closed-suction drain was placed in the retroperitoneal space as separate stab wounds were made in the abdomen for adequate removal of fluid and blood.

The inguinal canal was obliterated by closing the oblique and transversalis muscles in two layers using a #1 _____ (delayed absorbable) suture in a 'vest-over-pants' closure.

The inguinal incision was closed without tension with _____ suture and the groin specimen was sent to Pathology.

**Author's notes**

Transposition of the sartorius muscle is not described here as prophylactic antibiotics have essentially eliminated the need for this portion of the operation in regards to radical vulvectomy.

# Hemorrhoidal surgery

## Overview

There are several methods of removing hemorrhoids. Often the gynecological surgeon is faced with a patient with pelvic prolapse that includes hemorrhoids or even worse, rectal prolapse. The gynecologist that is able to correct these problems simultaneously with the pelvic defects will benefit the patient without having to refer the patient to a general surgeon for another operation. It is important to understand the classes of hemorrhoids (see Table) in order to be able to perform the best procedure.

## CLASS OF HEMORRHOIDS

| Class | Treatments |
| --- | --- |
| First degree | Diet, infrared coagulation, local and oral medicines (preparation, Anusol cream and/or suppositories, high fiber, etc.), sclerotherapy (injection of hyaluronic acid with water) |
| Second degree | Banding, sclerotherapy, or infrared coagulation |
| Third degree | Banding, hemorrhoidectomy, or PPH |
| Fourth degree | Hemorrhoidectomy or PPH |

## HEMORRHOIDECTOMY

### Technique

The patient was prepped and draped in the routine manner. The hemorrhoid was clamped at its base with a hemostat and excised. _____ (3-0 Vicryl or chromic) suture was utilized to reapproximate the incision in a _____ (continuous or interrupted) fashion. Hemostasis was excellent. A B & D suppository was placed in the rectum and lubricated packing with tag was placed in the rectum. The patient went to the PACU in excellent condition.

For deeper hemorrhoids, rubber band ligation or the Ferguson technique can be applied.

## PROCEDURE FOR PROLAPSED HEMORRHOIDS (PPH)

The procedure for prolapsed hemorrhoids (PPH) is a stapled hemorrhoidectomy that involves excising the prolapsed rectal mucosa above the dentate line and therefore pulling the hemorrhoids back up into the rectum.

### Indications

(1) Second-degree hemorrhoids after failure of rubber band ligature.
(2) Third- or second-degree hemorrhoids.
(3) Rectal mucosal prolapse.

### Contraindications

None

### Relative contraindications

(1) Acute thrombotic internal hemorrhoid(s).
(2) Previous perineal surgery.

### Specific needs

(1) Pre-op enema.
(2) Antibiotic prophylaxis optional.
(3) Anesthesia – general, regional, or other, including Versed (midazolam), Diprivan (propofol), and/or local.
(4) A PPH Procedural Set (Ethicon Endo-Surgery, Inc.).

### Advantages of PPH over other techniques

(1) Less pain.
(2) Quicker recovery.
(3) Shorter hospital stay.

### Disadvantages

(1) If too much tissue is drawn into the device, the rectal wall might be damaged.
(2) Short-term or long-term dysfunction of the internal sphincter muscles if the sphincter is stretched too much during the procedure.

## Technique

The patient was prepped and draped in the _____ (lithotomy, jack knife, etc.) position. Local anesthesia was injected into the rectal mucosa with a _____ (23–25) guage needle. Two finger dilatation of the rectum was performed with lubricated fingers. The dilator was placed into the rectum, removing the white portion while the assistant held the clear portion. Using the white anoscope, a purse-string suture was placed 4 cm above the dentate line using _____ (0–Prolene on a H-S or CT-2 needle). The needle was seen superficially during its entire placement. After one quadrant was sutured, the next quadrant was sutured, moving to the next using the obturator (white anoscope). The PPH instrument was placed into the purse-string suture until a pop was palpated then the purse-string suture was tied. The instrument hook was used to grasp the suture, then backward tension was placed on the purse-string suture and the instrument was closed.

The numbers could be seen on the instrument and the 4 cm mark was past the clear anoscope. The instrument was tightened all the way down, holding pressure for approximately 30 seconds as the instrument was steadied. The staples were applied then the closure device was turned a quarter-turn. The instrument was pulled out and the donut tissue of rectal mucosa with hemorrhoids was noted to be hemostatic. Gelfoam with antibiotic cream was applied to the inside of the rectum. The patient went to the PACU with Flagyl (mitronidazole) and instructions for stool softeners for 7–10 days.

# Hymenectomy

**Technique**

The patient was placed in the lithotomy position and, after adequate anesthesia, she was prepped and draped in the routine manner. The _____ (partially or fully) imperforate hymen was incised at 2, 4, 8, and 10 o'clock in a stellate fashion. The individual quadrants were then excised along the lateral wall of the vagina, being careful to avoid too close an excision to the vagina. The mucosal margins were reapproximated with fine 4-0 _____ (delayed absorbable) suture. Hemostasis and the result were excellent.

**Author's note**

Transcribe whether hematocolpos has already developed. Avoid D & C if hematocolpos has developed because of increased risk of perforating the thin overstretched uterine wall. Nothing more is needed unless the uterine mass does not regress within a few weeks. Dilatation may be needed if drainage from the uterus is unsatisfactory.

# Hypogastric artery ligation

**Important points/pearls**

Remember during obstetrical procedures that involve massive hemorrhage that the ovarian artery needs to be located above the pelvic brim because of the collateral blood supply. This artery also needs to be ligated but dissected free of the ovarian vein. A hemoclip is usually all that is necessary.

*Remember* to use a right-angle or Mixter clamp and pass it *lateral to medial* beneath the artery – hugging its surface. This protects the hypogastric vein. Doubly ligate – *DO NOT* transect. Palpate femoral pulses and identify the ureter before and after the procedure. Angiographic arterial embolization is an alternative using Gelfoam as small pledgets. MAST suits can be utilized while waiting if necessary.

**Author's notes**

Transcribe why a specific bleeding source was not found and/or the technical difficulty encountered in controlling hemorrhage during whatever difficult operative dissection was being performed, and then transcribe the following.

**Technique**

The peritoneum was opened on the lateral side of the common iliac artery near its bifurcation. The ureter was left attached to the medial peritoneal reflection so as to avoid disturbing its blood supply.

The posterior branch of the hypogastric artery was clearly identified, then the anterior division was dissected and mobilized free from the adjacent vein. Long vascular forceps and long vascular instruments were used for dissection. #0 _____ (silk) was passed *lateral to medial* around and beneath the artery, hugging its surface with a (an) _____ (right-angle or Adson clamp) and free-tied onto the artery. A second free-tie was placed distal to the initial ligature in similar fashion.

# Hysterectomy

## Overview

There are many new options in performing hysterectomy. An excellent gynecological surgeon should be able to perform all of these procedures and should be able to help the patient choose the correct hysterectomy for her condition. Minimally invasive procedures provide the benefits of decreased risks of muscle injury and postoperative incisional hernia. Factors such as obesity, history of prior abdominal surgery with possible adhesions, underlying medical conditions, the inability to safely visualize pelvic organs, or bleeding problems that are possibly foreseen during the operation are all reasons for choosing a particular type of hysterectomy.

---

**Important points/pearls**

- Know and be familiar with how to perform all the types of hysterectomy:

  | | |
  |---|---|
  | TAH | Total abdominal hysterectomy |
  | TLH | Total laparoscopic hysterectomy |
  | TVH | Total vaginal hysterectomy |
  | RH | Radical hysterectomy |
  | HALSH | Hand-assisted laparoscopic surgical hysterectomy |
  | LAVH | Laparoscopic-assisted vaginal hysterectomy |
  | LSH | Laparoscopic supracervical hysterectomy |
  | MIVH | Minimally invasive vaginal hysterectomy |

- Transcribe important points for the pre-op diagnosis:

  (1) If for DUB – make certain to transcribe if the bleeding is recurrent, severe, and unresponsive to HRT and curettage (how many times?)

  (2) Adenomyosis should be rarely, if ever, used as a pre-op diagnosis; it is a pathological diagnosis. Endometrial glands and stroma invading the myometrium is observed by either 1 per low power field, 2 per high power field, or to a depth of 3 mm.

  (3) Vaginal relaxation, prolapse, uterine descensus with or without SUI can be documented better if transcribed that ERT and Kegel exercises have failed or the patient is symptomatic.

  (4) Leiomyoma as a pre-op diagnosis can be enhanced by describing symptomatology (menorrhagia, metrorrhagia, discomfort,

---

etc.) Large size (greater than 12 cm) certainly provides better description and indication for hysterectomy.

(5) If hysterectomy is selected as treatment for PID, endometriosis, or another condition, make note of previously attempted conservative measures or explain why conservative measures were not an option.

(6) Criteria for hysterectomy include:

   (A) palpable myoma or concern to patient
   (B) excessive anemia (>8 days of anemia)
   (C) discomfort
   (D) rule out cervical cancer, anemia, medical diseases, and endometrial cancer prior to surgery

- Location of ureters: if an IVP is done prior to surgery, secondary to suspected mass effect or distortion, transcribe results during op report while locating the ureter. If there is any reason to suspect ureteral injury during any hysterectomy or to insure the integrity of the ureter during or after hysterectomy, indigo carmine can be given intravenously while the patient is still under general or regional anesthesia. The ureteral orifices would then be visualized via cystoscopy or cystotomy to have free flow of dye from each orifice.

- Antibiotics: infection is the most common complication of hysterectomy. Often, the prophylactic antibiotic that is given can be included in documentation of the op report. This demonstrates that the physician not only ordered it but also checked to see that it was given.

- Choice of hysterectomy: because of the advantages of vaginal hysterectomy over abdominal hysterectomy, if indicated and possible, the vaginal route should be the procedure of choice. MIVH is an excellent new option over TVH, LAVH, and others. Laparoscopic procedures can also still be considered prior to performing a TAH. If the surgeon is not comfortable or experienced with MIVH or TVH, a laparoscopic exam can be performed prior to vaginal surgery.

## *Determination of the route of hysterectomy*

Please see the flow chart (Figure) for determining the route of hysterectomy.

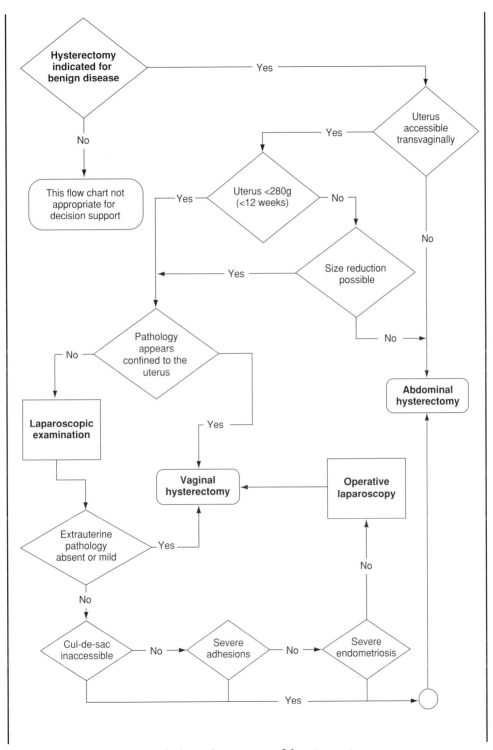

**Determining the route of hysterectomy**

- EUA: pelvic exam under anesthesia is often very helpful. Routine use and documentation of this manuever cannot be over-stated, especially when correlating operative findings with pelvic exam.
- Do not use excessive force to dissect the bladder flap away from the uterus or cervix – this can cause unnecessary blood loss or inadvertent entry into the bladder regardless of the route of hysterectomy.
- 'WATER UNDER THE BRIDGE': always palpate or examine the ureters prior to clamping the uterine vessels to make certain that these are not displaced by pathology. This is a very dangerous area for possible injury to the ureters.
- Keep clamps and cutting near the uterus in an almost 'rolling off' motion to avoid injury to lateral structures.
- Suspend the vaginal vault by incorporation of the cardinal, round, broad, and/or uterosacral ligaments to prevent future prolapse!
- Make sure the ovaries are retained against the pelvic side-walls and not adjacent to the vaginal cuff or the patient may subsequently complain of dyspareunia.
- If there is any doubt in regards to the integrity of the ureters, before the incision is closed, inject 5 ml of indigo carmine. Fill the bladder with approximately 200 ml of clear sterile saline and observe the ureteral orifices via cystoscopy. Within 3–5 minutes, the blue dye will be seen spurting from each orifice. (This can be performed routinely and easily if the hysterectomy is performed with the patient in Allen Universal stirrups as described in the 7th edn of TeLinde's *Operative Gynecology*. It can be done even easier if MIVH or TVH is performed with the patient in the candy cane stirrups.)

## TOTAL ABDOMINAL HYSTERECTOMY

### Technique

After satisfactory general anesthesia was obtained, an indwelling ure-thral catheter was placed and a careful pelvic examination under anes-thesia was performed, including the bimanual rectovaginal abdominal examination. Thorough Betadine vaginal preparation with particular emphasis on intravaginal cleansing of the vaginal fornices and also an abdominal prep was performed. Following the routine prep and drape, a _____ (type of incision) was carried out. This incision was carried down through the subcutaneous fascia, bringing about hemostasis with hemostats and electrocautery. Free ties were used as necessary. The fascia was entered with the scalpel blade and extended with Mayo scissors. The underlying rectus fascia and muscle layers were separated in the midline and the peritoneum was entered with two hemostats and scalpel blade. The peritoneum was extended with Metzenbaum scissors and following thorough washing of the powdered gloves with normal saline and standing on the patient's right side, the right hand was placed into the upper abdomen. After appropriate washings were obtained, the right kidney, liver, gallbladder, pancreas, stomach, left kidney, and para-aortic lymph nodes were palpated in sequence. (Findings are described.)

The _____ (O'Connor/O'Sullivan or Balfour) self-retaining retractor was placed into the abdominal cavity and opened for pelvic exposure. Adhesions were released so that the intestines could be placed in the upper abdomen and held there with _____ (wet lap packs or GYN bag).

The patient was placed in a modest Trendelenburg position and the round ligaments were bilaterally grasped with Kelly clamps near the uterine cornu, cut, and ligated with a 0- _____ (delayed absorbable) suture. The sutures were tagged bilaterally with a hemostat and left long.

The anterior leaves of the broad ligaments were incised to the point of reflection of the bladder peritoneum on the uterus. The avascular areas of the broad ligaments were located, incised, and the fallopian tubes and ovarian ligaments (infundibulopelvic ligaments if BSO is to be performed) were triply clamped as close as possible to the uterine corpus. Free ties using 0- _____ (delayed absorbable) sutures were placed as the second clamp of each cut pedicle bilaterally was removed. A 0- _____ (delayed absorbable) suture was placed in front of each of the first ligatures in the center of the pedicles beneath the remaining clamps and passing the free ends of the suture around the tips and heels of each clamp prior to tying. Both clamps were then removed.

The midline reflection of the bladder peritoneum onto the uterus was then freed by extending the incision into the anterior leaf of the broad ligament. The bladder was separated from the lower uterine segment and upper cervix by careful sharp dissection with the fascial fibers beneath the bladder wall. Mobilization of the bladder away from the cervix and upper anterior vaginal wall was performed. The posterior leaf of the broad ligament was then cut on either side parallel to the lateral side of the uterus. This was disected down to the point of origin on the uterosacral ligaments behind the cervix. Incising the anterior and posterior broad ligament peritoneum allowed the uterine vessels to be exposed and skeletonized with the Metzenbaum scissors bilaterally.

At this point the lower portions of the pelvic ureters were palpated as they coursed beneath the uterine arteries bilaterally, lateral to the internal cervical os bilaterally, and passed medially through the base of the broad ligament to enter the trigone of the bladder. With wide mobilization and displacement of the bladder base from the cervix, and with traction on the uterine corpus, the ureters were located lateral and inferior to the point of clamping of the uterine vessels. After completely exposing the uterine vessels by completely skeletonizing these vessels, they were then triply clamped bilaterally with curved _____ (Zephanelli, Ochsner, or Kocher) clamps. As the lowest clamp was placed initially, it was placed at the level of the internal cervical os and then also at right angles to the lower uterine segment. The other two clamps were placed above this first clamp. This was performed bilaterally. The vessels were cut with a scalpel between the upper and middle clamps and freed from the uterus by extending the incision around the tip of the middle clamp. Care was taken to avoid incising the tissue beyond the tip of the lowest clamp. Sutures were placed precisely in the angle of the incision and at the tip of the clamp, making certain that all vessels and the clamps were secured by ligature. This was performed bilaterally. The uterine vessels were doubly ligated with 0- _____ (delayed absorbable) suture with ligation of the tissue within the lowest clamp initially. As the first suture was tied bilaterally, the clamps were removed. As the second ligatures were placed and tied, the middle clamps were removed bilaterally. Following bilateral ligation of the uterine vessels, straight _____ (Zephanelli, Ochsner, or Ballentine) clamps were placed between the uterine vessels and bilateral sides of the uterus. The tissue was clamped bilaterally in the uppermost parts of the cardinal ligaments. This was then cut and suture ligated with 0- _____ (delayed absorbable) sutures. The uterus was pulled forward and upward to expose and stress the uterosacral ligaments posteriorly.

Each uterosacral ligament was clamped with a _____ (curved Zephanelli, Ochsner, or Ballentine clamp). Particular care was taken to avoid the pelvic portion of the ureter as it coursed along the base of the broad ligament. The uterosacral ligaments were then clamped, incised, and ligated with 0- _____ (delayed absorbable) sutures. Continued blunt and sharp dissection inferiorly in the center of the cul-de-sac between the ligated uterosacral ligaments developed a plane between the cervix and the vagina anteriorly and the anterior rectal wall posteriorly. At this point dissection of the bladder base away from the anterior vaginal wall was completed.

With the uterus under firm traction, the thumb and index finger from the same hand was made readily opposed below the cervix and further dissection of the base of the bladder anterior and the rectum posteriorly was accomplished. Particular attention to the pubovesicocervical fascia was then given as a small incision was made in the fascia anterior to the cervix just below the level of the internal cervical os and the ligated uterine vessels. As the edges of the fascia were retracted laterally, a pale avascular area of the anterior surface of the cervix and the vagina could be seen. The blunt end of scalpel was used in dissecting the loosened fibers of the pubovesicocervical fascia from the cervix. Dissection was continued with a sponge forcep until the fascia had been reflected far laterally off the anterior surface of the cervix and upper vagina. The whitish fascial plane of the vagina came into view. Dissection of the remaining portion of the cardinal ligaments was carried out by placing _____ (straight Zephanelli, Ochsner, or Ballentine) clamps inside the cut edges of the pubovesicocervical fascia. The lateral vaginal fornix was identified. The anterior and posterior walls of the vagina were clamped together at each lateral vaginal angle using a (an) _____ (Zephanelli, Ochsner, or Ballentine) clamp.

The uterus was removed by _____ [a circumferential incision made into the vagina as close to the cervix as possible using the curved _____ (Jorgenson) scissors] or a _____ (#170 or #200) polyroticulator was placed carefully under the cervix, clamped, and locked into place. The cervix was cut away from the vaginal cuff with the _____ (Jorgenson) scissors above the locked clamp. The polyroticulator was then unlocked and removed with absorbable staples, demonstrating good placement and good hemostasis. The entire cervix was removed with the uterine corpus.

*(If roticulator is not used, transcribe paragraph similar to this.)* _____ (Zephanelli, Ochsner, or Ballentine) clamps on the bilateral vaginal angles were replaced with transfixion Richardson sutures on each angle. The free margin of the vagina was then reefed with a continuous interlocking suture of 2-0 _____ (delayed absorbable) suture. *(If a drain is being placed through to the vagina, now is the time to transcribe it.*)* Hemostasis was maintained with figure-of-eight sutures, utilizing 2-0 _____ (delayed absorbable) suture in the vaginal vault.

Posterior and anterior culdoplasty was then performed. The right round ligament was then located and with the suture that had been placed on the round ligament, this hemostat was removed, and the suture was brought down into the vaginal corner suture. It was tied into place along with the suture from the cardinal ligament that had been left in place. These were reapproximated. The same procedure was performed on the left side as on the right side. Additional suspension of the vaginal vault was combined with peritonealization suture. In this technique, use of a continuous 0- _____ (delayed absorbable) suture was used to pierce the vaginal wall and it was passed through the ligated pedicle of the angle of the vagina and the free margin of the cardinal ligament, staying distal to the original cardinal ligament ligature. The suture was then passed through the anterior bladder peritoneum near the round ligament. The suture was continued through the free margin of the round ligament and the remaining edge of the anterior leaf of the broad ligament incorporating the free margin of the utero-ovarian ligament. It was continued posteriorly along the cut edge of the posterior leaf of the broad ligament incorporating the uterosacral ligament. This suture finally pierced the posterior edge of the vaginal wall near the midline. The ligatures were all tied firmly in the midline. The same procedure was performed on the left side as was performed on the right, and this accomplished vaginal vault suspension and peritonealization on each side. The tip of the broad ligament was closed separately with a purse-string suture of 3-0 _____ (delayed absorbable) suture and the free margin of the pedicle was buried beneath the peritoneum, allowing the ovaries to be retained high against the pelvic wall and not anchored to the vaginal vault. This was performed bilaterally.

Peritonealization was completed by suturing the bladder peritoneum to the cul-de-sac peritoneum with 3-0 _____ (delayed absorbable) suture. This suture was initiated near the angle of the vagina where the anterior peritoneum was pierced and the peritoneum over the round ligament and infundibulopelvic ligament was picked up before the cul-de-sac peritoneum was sutured. The suture was tied and then continued to the opposite angle of the vagina as a continuous suture approximating the bladder and cul-de-sac peritoneum. The pelvis was inspected and thoroughly irrigated with normal saline solution. The normal saline was suctioned off with the suction tip and the lap pads and the self-retaining retractor was removed.

The peritoneum was closed in a continuous fashion, utilizing 2-0 _____ in a three-point stitch to avert the cut peritoneal edges and to make the intraperitoneal suture line as smooth as possible. Hemostasis was judged to be excellent and the muscles were reapproximated in the midline with interrupted sutures of 2-0 _____ . The fascial edges were approximated with single #1 _____ suture, utilizing a modification of the far/near, near/far suture method. Subcutaneous fat was approximated with interrupted sutures of 3-0 _____ suture following thorough irrigation of this area. The skin was closed with a _____ (4-0 Vicryl subcuticular stitch). Following cleansing of the skin, a (Telfa and bandage) were applied with routine dressing. Instrument, lap, needle, and sponge counts were all correct. The patient was removed to the Recovery Room in stable condition.

---

**Author's notes**

*If a polyroticulator was *not* used, transcribe. If a roticulator was used, omit paragraph 10. If a drain was placed through to the vagina, it must be described.

## TOTAL ABDOMINAL HYSTERECTOMY WITH BILATERAL SALPINGO-OOPHORECTOMY (BRIEF FORM STYLE)

### Technique

The patient was prepped and draped in the usual manner with the legs placed in Allen Universal stirrups. Examination under anesthesia was performed under sterile conditions following thorough Betadine prep. A Foley catheter was placed into the urethral orifice until urine was obtained and the catheter was left in place. The surgical prep and drape was completed and then gloves and gown were changed. A lower abdominal transverse Maylard incision was performed and carried down through the subcutaneous tissue to the fascia. Hemostasis was performed using hemostats and electrocautery. The fascia was entered with scalpel blade and extended with Mayo scissors. The underlying rectus fascia and muscle layer was separated in the midline and the peritoneum was entered with two hemostats and Metzenbaum scissors. The incision was extended with Metzenbaum scissors following washing of the gloves in the splash basin. Standing on the patient's right side, the abdominal and peritoneal washings were obtained with catheter. The upper abdomen was explored, including the right liver, kidney, gallbladder, pancreas, stomach, left kidney, and periaortic lymph nodes. The findings were normal. The Bookwalter self-retaining retractor was placed into the abdomen with lap-packs to provide adequate exposure.

Round ligaments were bilaterally clamped, cut, and suture ligated using curved Ochsner clamps and _____ (#2-0, delayed absorbable) suture. The anterior leaves of the broad ligaments were then entered to the point of reflection on the bladder and the avascular portion of the broad ligament was incised with scissors, thus making a window in the broad ligament bilaterally. After fully assessing the condition of the ovaries, it was decided that bilateral salpingo-oophorectomy would be in the best interest of this patient. Infundibulopelvic ligaments were bilaterally triply clamped, cut, and suture-ligated with both a free-tie and a suture ligature. The uterine vessels were exposed and the lower portion of the pelvic ureters were palpated as each coursed beneath the uterine arteries bilaterally, lateral to the internal cervical os bilaterally, passing medially through the base of the broad ligament until each entered the trigone of the bladder. With wide mobilization, displacement of the bladder base from the cervix using a sponge stick and with traction on the uterine corpus, the ureters were located lateral and inferior to the point of clamping the uterine vessels. The uterine vessels were triply clamped bilaterally with curved Ochsner clamps. The clamps had been placed at the level of the internal cervical os at right angles to the lower uterine segment. The other two clamps were placed above the first clamp. This was performed bilaterally.

The uterine vessels were cut with scalpel blade between the upper and middle clamps and freed from the uterus by extending the incision around the tip of the middle clamp. Care was taken to avoid incising the tissue beyond the tip of the lowest clamp. The sutures were placed precisely at an angle of the incision and at the tip of the clamp, making certain that all vessels and clamp were secured by ligature. This was performed bilaterally.

The uterine vessels were then doubly ligated with _____ (0-delayed absorbable) suture bilaterally. The clamps were removed and then straight Ballentine clamps were placed between the uterine vessels and the ligated uterine vessels dropped laterally away from the uterus bilaterally. The cardinal ligaments were bilaterally clamped and suture-ligated with _____ (0-delayed absorbable) suture. Ballentine clamps were used to perform further isolation of the uterosacral ligaments, as these were clamped, cut, and suture-ligated with _____ (0-delayed absorbable) suture bilaterally. Further clamping, cutting, and suture-ligating of the uterosacral ligaments on the bilateral sides of the uterus was performed, taking care to avoid the pelvic portions of the ureters, as each coursed along the base of the broad ligament.

The bladder base was dissected away from the anterior vaginal wall, using both sharp and blunt dissection. With the uterus under firm traction and the thumb and index finger from the same hand made readily opposed below the cervix, further dissection was performed along the base of the bladder anterior and posterior along the rectum. Particular attention to the pubovesicocervical fascia was made as the _____ (#170 polyreticulator) was placed under the cervix. The reticulator was applied and staples clamped into place. As the reticulator was locked and staples applied, the Jorgenson scissors were then used to dissect the cervix away from the vaginal cuff. The entire cervix was removed from the operative field and then entire uterus, cervix, and bilateral ovaries and tubes were sent to Pathology.

Sutures on the round ligaments and uterosacral and cardinal ligaments were reapproximated along the corner of the vaginal cuff to provide support to the new pelvic floor. The peritoneum was then closed over the bladder cuff with _____ (2-0 delayed absorbable) suture. The entire area was irrigated thoroughly prior to closing the bladder cuff and hemostasis was judged to be excellent.

The peritoneum was closed with _____ (2-0 delayed absorbable) suture in a continuous fashion. The muscle layer was closed in an interrupted fashion with (0-delayed absorbable) suture. The fascia was closed with _____ (#1-delayed absorbable) suture in a continuous fashion. Each layer was irrigated thoroughly prior to closure. The subcutaneous tissue was closed with _____ (3-0 plain) suture in a continuous fashion. The skin was closed with skin staples. The incision was wiped clean with a wet lap–dry lap and bandage was applied. The patient tolerated the procedure very well.

Cystoscopy was not performed because ureters were bilaterally palpated and visualized to be intact and very functional during and after the procedure.

## RADICAL HYSTERECTOMY

Exploratory laparotomy; bilateral salpingo-oophorectomy; periaortic and pelvic lymphadenectomies bilateral; and lysis of adhesions are included in this transcription for completeness.

### Technique

The patient was placed in modified dorsolithotomy position after IVCC booties had been connected, and general anesthesia had been induced. A Foley catheter was inserted. She was placed supine and after exam under anesthesia had been carried out, the findings of which are noted above, she was then prepped and draped in a sterile fashion. The abdominal cavity was opened through midline vertical incision extending from symphysis to umbilicus. On entry, exploration was carried out, findings noted above. The upper abdominal viscera were all palpated _____ (normal).

Attention was turned to the pelvis after a self-retaining retractor had been placed and the bowels packed away superiorly. The uterus was grasped with large Kelly clamps bilaterally and elevated. Round ligaments were divided using _____ (an LDS $CO_2$-powered device). The vesicouterine reflection was sharply incised transversely. The infundibulopelvic ligaments were isolated and when the ureters were seen to be clear and free, the infundibulopelvic ligaments were divided with _____ (an LDS $CO_2$-powered device). Additional _____ (0 chromic ties) were placed on these pedicles. Bilaterally, the perivesical and perirectal spaces were opened down to the levator muscles. The course of the distal obliterated hypogastric arteries bilaterally was identified and these vessels skeletonized; thereby, they were able to be retracted laterally out of harm's way. All the pelvic and periaortic nodal areas were palpated and there was no adenopathy appreciated.

First on the right, the origin of the uterine vessels was identified; the web was carefully retracted so as to expose it satisfactorily. The ureter reflected medial out of harm's way and the structures of the web, including the uterine vessels, were taken at their origin, and/or insertion into the hypogastric artery or vein, respectively. All this was a clip-and-cut technique. It was carried out down to the level of the levator muscles. An identical procedure was repeated on the opposite side.

The course of the right ureter was identified, it was dissected off the peritoneal reflection posteriorly, and was skeletonized down to its entry into the cardinal ureteric tunnel. It was unroofed using _____ (Lahey clamps). The specimen side was clamped and the patient side was tied with _____ (00 chromic). The ureter was dissected all the way down to its splaying into the bladder base. An identical procedure was repeated on the opposite side.

The rectovaginal septum was opened with sharp dissection and the rectum pushed away posteriorly. The ureterosacral ligaments bilaterally were taken near their insertion into the bony pelvic wall with _____ (Heaney clamps) using a clamp, cut, and Heaney ligature _____ (0 chromic) technique. Laterally parametrial pedicles were developed with Heaney clamps. The entire surgical specimen consisting of cervix and corpus uteri, as well as both tubes and ovaries, parametrium, paracolpos, and upper one-third of the vagina was placed on additional further upward traction. The ureters were reflected laterally out of harm's way, the rectum posteriorly and the bladder anteriorly. Kidney pedicle C-clamps were placed. Below these, Heaney clamps were placed and a transverse incision freed the above-mentioned surgical specimen. Modified Aldridge angle sutures were placed in the lateral vaginal angles, and the posterior cuff was run in continuity to the parietal peritoneum of the colon, the anterior cuff was run in continuity with the parietal peritoneum overlying the bladder, all with _____ (0 chromic). Then a rainbow arcade stitch was placed from side-to-side, thus recreating the upper one-third of the vagina. The pelvis was irrigated and hemostasis was noted to be satisfactory.

Bilateral aortic and pelvic lymphadenectomy was then accomplished from just below the level of the renal vessels down to the level of the circumflex iliac veins into the floor of the obturator fossa below the level of the obturator nerves bilaterally. Great care was taken at all times to avoid injury to the ureters, the vessels, and the nerves in the operated areas. Nodal material was labeled as to site of origin and was removed using a clip-and-cut technique. Bilaterally, drains were placed in the retroperitoneal areas, the pelvis was irrigated, and hemostasis noted to be satisfactory. Exit sites of the peritoneal drains were secured on the anterior abdominal wall with box-type stitches.

One ampule of indigo carmine was injected along with a fluid bolus. There was a prompt clearing of the dye through the kidneys with ureters found to peristalsis normally. There was no evidence of extravasation of the blue urine from either ureter or the bladder.

Bowels were returned to an anatomical position. Sponge, instrument, and needle count was reported as correct times two. The abdominal wall was closed with modified Smead–Jones figure-of-eight _____ (#1 Prolene). The subcutaneous layer was irrigated with Betadine, and saline. Skin closure was achieved with _____ (metallic clips). Dry, pressure dressing was placed on the wound. The patient tolerated the operative procedure well and was transferred to the Recovery Room in satisfactory condition.

## Acknowledgment

This transcription was contributed by Dr Charles H. Pippitt, then reviewed and edited by Dr John E. Turrentine.

## TOTAL LAPAROSCOPIC HYSTERECTOMY

### Specific needs

(1)  3 Trocars
(2)  Laparoscopic tissue manipulator
(3)  5 mm LCS (Harmonic ACE)
(4)  Suturing graspers
(5)  Tissue extractor

### Important tips

In paragraph 6, a detailed description of using a laparoscopic suturing technique is given. This much detail is not necessary in transcription. It is only described here for teaching purposes. All gynecological-laparoscopic surgeons should be adept in laparoscopic suturing techniques.

### Technique

After the patient was anesthetized, the patient's legs were placed in Allen stirrups and a pelvic examination was performed under anesthesia. The vagina was prepped with _____ (Betadine or Hibiclens). The patient's abdomen was then prepped with _____ (Betadine or Hibiclens), with special attention around the umbilicus. The patient was then draped with sterile leggings and laparoscopic drapes.

A small incision was carried out through the umbilicus using a #11 blade scalpel. Using hemostats and Mayo scissors, dissection was down to the fascia, at which time the fascia was incised carefully and each side of the incision picked up with forceps (with teeth). _____ (#2–0 Vicryl) suture with a Uro-6 needle was placed in the fascia on each side of the incision. Two hemostats were then used to pick up the peritoneum. This was carefully incised in an attempt to avoid underlying viscera. After identifying the abdominal cavity, the trocar was placed inside the abdomen and the two sutures were used to hold it in place. (*As an alternative, an Ethicon non-traumatic clear bladeless 10/12 handled, 10/12 non-handled, or 5 mm non-handled bladeless trocar – short or long – can be used to enter the peritoneum).* The $CO_2$ hose was attached to the trocar and approximately 2.5 liters of $CO_2$ were insufflated into the abdomen. The camera was then attached to the top of the trocar lens.

After visualizing the placement of the two other abdominal trocars via monitor, a laparoscopic tissue manipulator was placed through the _____ (left or right) lower abdominal trocar. The Harmonic ACE was placed through the other trocar. Stabilizing the uterus with the manipulator, the round ligaments were clamped, using minimum coagulation, and clipped. The uterus was relaxed and the ACE was not moved. After the round ligaments were bilaterally bisected, an endo-peanut was used to dissect the bladder away from the lower uterine segment and anterior vaginal mucosa. The broad ligaments were clamped and clipped with the ACE bilaterally using minimum coagulation. The bilateral uterine arteries were also clamped and cut using minimum coagulation, being very careful to keep the ACE in one place at a 90° angle to the vessels.

Using a sponge stick in the vagina, the anterior and posterior colpotomies were carried out and the vagina was packed with _____ (a wet Operating Room towel or balloon packer) to prevent $CO_2$ leakage. The Harmonic ACE was continually used in conjunction with the uterine manipulator to clamp, clip, and hit minimal coagulation. Care was taken to stay medial to the uterine and cardinal ligaments *(just as is done when using two clamps in a TAH but using the ACE)*.

Eventually, once the uterus was removed from its attachments, it was removed using the endopouch retriever. *(If the uterus is too large to remove in this manner, it may be morcellated during the procedure after the uterine arteries are bisected by using the laparoscopic morcellator)*.

The anterior and posterior colpotomies are then connected using _____ (3–0 Monocryl on an SH taper needle or a CT-1 Vicryl suture). After cutting a 5–6 inch piece of suture attached to a self-righting needle holder (SRNH) and placing these through the laparoscopic sleeve, the suture was grasped close to the needle. The German needle holder (GNH) was placed through the other sleeve. With the tip of the GNH, the tip of the needle was gently grasped from the side and the SRNH was released. From a perpendicular angle, with the SRNH, the needle was grasped one-third of the distance from its swedge end and then the GNH was released. Full-thickness bites were taken using an SRNH, using the tip of the needle perpendicular to the surface and, through rotation of the wrist, rotating the needle through the tissue. The protruding tip of the needle is grasped with the GNH, and the SRNH is released. The needle is stabilized with the non-dominant hand. The needle is regrasped with the SRNH and, following the curve of the needle, the wrist is rotated to pull suture through the tissue. Approximately 1 inch of suture tail is left. The needle is rotated so that the suture end is toward the GNH. The suture is looped around the tip of the GNH twice and the GNH is advanced to grasp the tail. The SRNH is pulled to slide the loops off the GNH and the loop is tightened. The GNH is moved slightly in the opposite direction to assist in this maneuver. The suture tail is released. The needle is passed to the GNH, grasping it at the tip and pointing the suture end toward the SRNH. The suture is wrapped once around the SRNH, grasping the tail with the SRNH, and both holders equally pulled to tighten the knot. Both ends of the suture were handed to the GNH, the SRNH was removed and replaced with scissors. The scissors were used to cut the suture, then the suture and needle were removed from the GNH port. An anterior modified Richardson suturing technique was used to bring the anterior and posterior vaginal cuff together to be reapproximated.

Irrigation was then carried out with the laparoscopic irrigator. The uterine stumps *(and I-P stumps if adnexa was removed)* were carefully checked. There appeared to be no injury to viscera. All instruments, needles, sponges, peanuts, and towels were counted and found to be correct. All instruments were removed from the abdomen under visualization. Hemostasis was excellent. Fascia and skin were closed with _____ (0 Vicryl and 5-0 Vicryl). These areas were cleaned and Band-Aids applied. _____ (Towel or balloon device) was removed from the vagina. The patient was stable and went to the PACU in excellent condition.

## TOTAL VAGINAL HYSTERECTOMY (WITH SUSPENSION OF THE VAGINAL VAULT)

### Technique

After the patient was anesthetized, a pelvic examination was carried out under anesthesia. (Findings may be transcribed.) After proper scrub, the patient was placed in the dorsolithotomy position with the hips located at the edge of the table so that a weighted speculum could swing free, the vulva, perineum, and vagina were thoroughly washed with _____ (Betadine or Hibiclens). The bladder was emptied with a catheter and clamped. With the cervix exposed, it was grasped with a tenaculum and pulled strongly into view. 10 ml of dilute Neo-Synephrine solution (1:200 000) was injected into the anterior and posterior vaginal fornices.

A semilunar incision was made through the mucosa of the vaginal fornix just above the portio but below the attachment of the bladder. The bladder was freed from the anterior surface of the uterus by sharp dissection up to the plica vesicouterinea. After the loose areolar plane was entered and the fascial attachments were excised beneath the bladder with the curved Mayo scissors, the dissection was completed with the finger covered with gauze. The free peritoneal fold was identified and incised. A narrow-bladed retractor was inserted into the peritoneal cavity to hold the bladder and the ureters forward. Following this entry into the anterior cul-de-sac, the cervix was pulled strongly forward and a semilunar incision was made through the vaginal mucosa at the height of the posterior fornix and the anterior and posterior incisions were joined on each side of the cervix. Care was taken to avoid injury to the rectum. After cutting through the mucosa, the loose areolar plane was entered and the space was developed by sharp dissection until the peritoneum was visible. The cul-de-sac was explored and a narrow right-angle retractor was introduced. The peritoneal reflection was then excised under direct vision. Pushing back the mucosa, the peritoneum exposed the base of the cardinal ligaments.

The base of the cardinal ligament was clamped separately by a _____ (Zephanelli or Heaney) clamp and was then cut on the uterine side and the clamp was replaced by a fixation suture using #1 _____ (delayed absorbable) suture. Next the uterosacral ligament was clamped with a Heaney clamp, excised, and transfixed with a similar suture. The ligated pedicle was held for later placation by an identifying hemostat and this would be used later during a vaginal vault suspension. The retractor was placed in both the anterior and posterior cul-de-sac to allow excellent exposure of the left broad ligament while displacing the bladder, ureter, and rectum. After the base of the cardinal ligament and left uterosacral ligament were separately cut and ligated, the uterine vessels could be seen.

The vessels were similarly clamped, cut, but replaced by a nontransfixion suture using a #1 _____ (delayed absorbable) suture. In successive similar steps, the broad ligament on the left was disposed of as high as possible, picking up the anterior peritoneum above the uterine vessels with each successive pedicle.

When further progress on the left could not be made, the retractors were shifted to the right of the patient and the right cardinal ligament was clamped, cut, and ligated in similar fashion. The uterosacral ligament was clamped, excised, and transfixed separately and the ligature was held with a hemostat. In similar steps on the right the uterine vessels were ligated but not transfixed and the right broad ligament was severed from the uterus as high as exposure allowed. After the broad ligaments had been excised as high as possible on each side of the uterine body, the cervix was pulled superiorly.

The uterine body then presented itself at the posterior opening, where it was grasped by a Lahey clamp. This was partially pulled outside the introitus. The upper portion of the broad ligament, the uterine end of the tube, and the suspensory ligament of the ovary and the round ligament on the left side were now identified and were carefully inspected. These structures were incorporated into the cornual portion of the broad ligament, which was clamped, cut, and doubly ligated. This was performed with a free tie to occlude the vascular pedicle and then it was transfixed with a stay suture placed on the outside of the previous ligature. The outer ligature on the pedicle from the tip of the broad ligament was held with a Kelly clamp to identify this ligament at the time of peritonealization and suspension of the vaginal vault. After the left side of the uterus was freed, the right cornual region was clamped, excised, and ligated by a similar technique.

The uterus was removed and inspected to see whether any pathological process existed and the findings can be seen as above. After the uterus was removed, a small wet laparotomy pack was held by a small clamp.

Suspension of the vaginal vault was performed by a continuous suture utilizing #1 _____ (delayed absorbable) suture placed through the lateral vaginal wall and adjacent to the peritoneum. The suture was continued through the tip of the broad ligament, cardinal ligament, and uterosacral ligament before returning through the vaginal wall. After suspension was completed on both sides, the patient culdoplasty suture was passed through the uterosacral ligament, cul-de-sac, peritoneum, and opposite ligament, which was the internal suture. The second suture was placed slightly higher. External culdoplasty sutures were placed through the posterior fornix and passed through each uterosacral ligament before returning through cul-de-sac, peritoneum, and posterior fornix. A purse-string suture was used to encircle the peritoneal surface as the highest internal suture utilizing 0 _____ (delayed absorbable) suture. The peritoneal suture was placed in a manner in which the vascular pedicles were in an extraperitoneal position so as to avoid intraperitoneal bleeding.

The suspension sutures in the lateral vaginal angles were tied and the uterosacral plication sutures were now tied both internally and in the posterior fornix. The purse-string suture was then tied and found to be adequately closed in that a finger could not be admitted. Transverse closure of the vaginal vault was then performed with figure-of-eight sutures utilizing 0 Vicryl. _____ inch iodoform packing was then placed in the vagina. Estimated blood loss was _____. Instruments, needle, sponge, and lap counts were all correct. The patient went to the PACU in excellent condition.

## TOTAL VAGINAL HYSTERECTOMY (WITH LASH INCISION AND MORCELLATION)

---

**Pearl**

Morcellation is relatively safe once the uterine arteries have been secured and location of the ureter is known.

---

**Technique**

After the patient was anesthetized, a pelvic examination was carried out under anesthesia. (Findings may be transcribed.) After proper scrub, the patient was placed in the dorsolithotomy position with the hips located at the edge of the table so that a weighted speculum could swing free, and the vulva, perineum, and vagina were thoroughly washed with _____. The bladder was emptied with a catheter and clamped. With the cervix exposed, it was grasped with a tenaculum and pulled strongly into view.

An incision around the cervix with the Bovie unit was made through the mucosa of the vaginal fornix just above the portio but below the attachment of the bladder and through the vaginal mucosa at the height of the posterior fornix. Dissection was performed until the peritoneal fold was identified; then this area was incised and a narrow-bladed retractor was inserted. The posterior peritoneum was then excised under direct vision and the cul-de-sac was explored and a narrow right-angle retractor was introduced. Pushing back the mucosa, the peritoneum exposed the base of the cardinal ligaments.

The bases of the cardinal ligaments were clamped separately by _____ (Zephanelli or Heaney) clamps, cut and replaced by fixation sutures using #1 _____ (delayed absorbable) suture. Next, the uterosacral ligaments were clamped, excised, and transfixed with a similar suture. The ligated pedicles were held for later plication by identifying hemostats.

The uterine vessels were similarly clamped, cut, but replaced by non-transfixion sutures using a #1_____ (delayed absorbable) suture. In successive similar steps, the broad ligaments bilaterally were disposed of as high as possible, picking up the anterior peritoneum above the uterine vessels with each successive pedicle.

It was noted, however, that the uterine body was too large to present itself at the introitus, and therefore a lash incision was carried out along both sides of the lower uterine segment in an attempt to invert the uterus. Completion of the operation using only this method was unsuccessful, and therefore morcellation was performed in that the cervix and lower uterine segment was amputated first followed by several other portions of myometria until there was enough exposure in order to grasp the remaining uterus with a _____ (long Lahey or double or tooth tenaculum). *(Morcellation may also be used if that portion of the uterus is outside the vagina. It is NOT recommended to use the morcellator inside the vagina unless there is excellent visibility and it can be made certain that the vagina CANNOT come in contact with the morcellator, as this could cause SERIOUS laceration and damage to the vagina.)*

The remaining uterus was partially pulled outside the introitus. The upper portions of the broad ligaments, the uterine ends of the tubes, and the suspensory ligaments of the ovaries and the round ligaments on both sides were now identified and were carefully inspected. These structures were incorporated into the cornual portions of the broad ligaments, which were clamped, cut, and doubly ligated. This was performed with free ties to occlude the vascular pedicles, and these were transfixed with stay sutures placed on the outside of the previous ligatures. The outer ligatures on the pedicles from the tips of the broad ligaments were held with Kelly clamps to identify these ligaments at the time of peritonealization and suspension of the vaginal vault.

The uterus, having been removed in portions, was examined for gross pathology. *(Describe findings here or in pretechnique note.)* After the uterus was removed, a small wet laparotomy pack was held by a small clamp.

Suspension of the vaginal vault was performed by a continuous suture utilizing #1 _____ (delayed absorbable) suture placed through the lateral vaginal wall and adjacent to the peritoneum. The suspension sutures in the lateral vaginal angles were tied and the uterosacral plication sutures were now tied both internally and in the posterior fornix. The purse-string suture was then tied and found to be adequately closed in that a finger could not be admitted.

Transverse closure of the vaginal vault was then performed with figure-of-eight sutures utilizing 0 Vicryl. _____ inch iodoform packing was then placed in the vagina. Estimated blood loss was _____. Instruments, needle, sponge, and lap counts were all correct.

## HAND-ASSISTED LAPAROSCOPIC HYSTERECTOMY

**Pearls**

- HALS (hand-assisted laparoscopic surgery) was first used in 1993 for a splenectomy. Since that time, adrenalectomy, gastrectomies, nephrectomies, colectomies, and hysterectomies have been done this way.

- Advantages of HALS include helping restore hand–eye coordination (3D), direct tactile sensation, improved exposure and traction, shortens dissection maneuvers/times, bleeding control, large mass mobility and removal, and fewer trocars. It utilizes the ideal surgical tool – the human hand.
- Disadvantages of HALS are that it requires a 6 cm+ incision (surgeon's glove size −1 cm), the hand can be in the way of trocar placement, and there are increased risks of fatigue and spasm.
- HALS is most useful with large fibroids (16–28 weeks' size) that are incarcerated, calcified, or if two morcellators are to be used (two are usually needed if the fibroid is over 400 g). HALS is helpful if there are posterior fibroids, obtaining a good two-layer closure, and ease of enucleation and morcellation.
- HALS is also useful in approaching adnexal masses. One can minimize spills, complete cystectomy, dissect endometrioma away from the pelvic wall, deal with tough PID cases, and dissect 8 cm masses at 16–18 weeks' gestation via gentle manipulation.

**Specific needs**

(1) 30° 5 mm laparoscope and video
(2) Lap Disc
(3) Suction irrigator-aspirator
(4) 5 mm Harmonic Shears (ACE) (Ethicon Endo-Surgery, Inc.)
(5) 5 mm graspers
(6) Two 5 mm bladeless trocars
(7) Scalpel, Foley, towel clamps, etc. . . .

**Technique**

The patient was prepped and draped in the usual manner for a laparoscopic procedure. A small incision was carried out to the left of the umbilicus. The incision was made _____ (1 cm smaller than the surgeon's glove size) long. The incision was made into the peritoneum. Stay sutures were placed into the peritoneum and fascia. The lap disc was inserted with one hand while the other hand was used to pull up the stay sutures in the abdominal wall. The other stay suture was then lifted and the reversed portion of the flexible ring was slowly pushed into the abdominal cavity through the anterior wall and carefully expanded. It was made certain that the flexible ring fully contacted the anterior abdominal wall and was seated securely with no viscera inadvertently between the ring and peritoneum. *(The endoscope can be used to facilitate proper placement.)* The iris valve was shut by rotating the upper ring clockwise. The upper and lower rings were pressed and rotated together. The upper ring was slightly twisted counterclockwise to lock the gears shut. Once the insufflation trocar was inserted into the abdominal cavity, the iris valve was dilated for handoscopy. By rotating the upper ring clockwise with a half-rotation, the iris valve was easily adjusted to fit _____ (name of surgeon) wrist. The hand, with the aid of sterile lubricant, could then be easily inserted and removed.

At this point, using the hand to assist the surgery, the _____ TLH, LAVH, LSH, and/or myomectomy, adrenalectomy, or other procedure is transcribed in routine manner.

## LAPAROSCOPIC-ASSISTED VAGINAL HYSTERECTOMY (WITH BSO)

### Specific needs

(1)  Three 5 mm trocars
(2)  5 mm laparoscope
(3)  One LCS curve blade or Harmonic ACE
(4)  5 mm single-tooth uterine manipulator or laparoscopic manipulator
(5)  Vaginal sponge stick.

---

**Pearl**

During LAVH, the uterine vessels are secured VAGINALLY. In contrast, during TLH or LSH, the uterine vessels are secured ABDOMINALLY!!!

---

**Technique**

The patient was prepped and draped with Betadine in the lithotomy position. The weighted speculum was placed into the vagina and a single-tooth tenaculum was utilized on the anterior lip of the cervix. The tenaculum was placed into the intrauterine cavity and the uterus was stabilized. Ureteral catheters were bilaterally placed cystoscopically (*this can be done if ureters are not dissected into view laparoscopically*). The single-tooth tenaculum was removed and all retractors removed. A catheter was placed with Foley bag, and attention was placed on the abdomen. Gloves were changed. A small subumbilical incision was carried out and a Surgiport Verres needle was placed in the routine manner. Placement was checked by the hanging drop method, the syringe method, gas pressure register method, and the bubble method. Pneumoperitoneum of approximately 3 liters of $CO_2$ was established and the laparoscopic _____ (5 mm) trocar was placed in the routine manner, withdrawing the trocar and listening for sound of escaping gas for confirmation of proper location. Video fiberoptics were connected and the videoscope was gently inserted under direct video laparoscopic visualization. Trendelenburg position was increased and approximately 1.5 liters more of gas was allowed into the abdomen to better displace the viscera so as to easily visualize the pelvic organs. *(Describe gross pathology.)* The 5 mm trocar incisions were made in the lower abdomen and 5 mm laparoscopic trocars were placed, visualizing the placement via video camera during the entire procedure. A small midline incision was carried out approximately 5–10 cm below the umbilicus and another 5 mm trocar was placed through this incision under direct video laparoscopic visualization. There appeared to be no complications during placement of extra trocars. A 5 mm laparoscopic grasper was utilized to lift the right ovary and fallopian tube toward the midline. Endogage was secured to determine whether a 3.5 or 3 V staple size should be used. Through the 5 mm trocar sleeve, the Harmonic Ace was utilized to transect the interphalangeal (IP) ligament. The area was checked for hemostasis. *(The Harmonic ACE can be used to coagulate and transect the IP ligaments but care must be taken to keep the ACE still and at 90° angles, otherwise a 10/12 trocar should be used with a GIA-30 stapler.)* The round and broad ligaments were also clamped, coagulated, and transected with the Harmonic ACE and manipulated so that the grasper held the ovary and fallopian tube in place, in order to make placement easy. Following the removal of the right ovary and tube, a 5 mm grasper was placed through one port and an endo pouch through the other port. The ovary and tube were pulled up through the _____ (5 mm) sleeve, grasped with a Kelly clamp on the outside of the abdomen, and morcellated appropriately to remove the tissue through the small incision. The same procedure was performed on the left side, as was on the right, in that the 5 mm laparoscopic grasper was used to manipulate the left ovary and tube in order to place the Harmonic ACE through the 5 mm sleeve so as to clamp, coagulate, and cut the left infundibulopelvic ligament at 90° angles. The ovary and tube were then removed through the _____ (5 mm) sleeve. The area was found to be hemostatic. There appeared to be no injury to any abdominal viscera. The round and broad ligaments were then bilaterally clamped and cut using the Harmonic ACE through the 5 mm sleeve and then the bladder flap was developed using the endo peanut and laparoscopic scissors and Harmonic ACE. The flap was created using laparoscopic scissors or contact minimal ACE technique, thus exposing the anterior cul-de-sac. The ureteral catheters were continually moved and palpated so as to identify the ureters.

At this point, attention was directed to the vagina. Pneumoperitoneum was maintained until anterior colpotomy was performed. Posterior colpotomy was also completed. Uterosacral and cardinal ligaments were bilaterally clamped, cut, and ligated using _____ (Zephanelli or Heaney clamps) and _____ (2-0 delayed absorbable suture). Uterine vessels were then bilaterally clamped with _____ (Zephanelli or Heaney clamps), cut with Mayo scissors, and ligated with _____ (2-0 Vicryl) suture, and the uterus was removed. Vaginal cuff was reapproximated with _____ (0-delayed absorbable) suture in hemostatic fashion. Pneumoperitoneum was re-established, and vaginal cuff and suture lines were inspected for tissue approximation and hemostasis. Irrigator was used as necessary. All instrumentation was then removed and incisions reapproximated with _____ (0 Vicryl and 5-0 Vicryl) suture. Neosporin and bandages were applied over incisions. All instrument, needle, and sponge counts were correct. The patient went to the PACU in excellent condition.

## LAPAROSCOPIC SUPRACERVICAL HYSTERECTOMY

### Important points

The re-emergence of the subtotal hysterectomy came about with the increasing use of laparoscopic hysterectomies. Prior to 1960, leaving the cervix during hysterectomy was secondary to increased surgical risk (increased infection, injury to ureter, and difficulty of surgery). Presently, these are some of the same reasons. However, Dr Steven McCarus of Orlando, Florida has been an innovator in taking a second look at the subtotal or laparoscopic supracervical hysterectomy (LSH).

To sum up Dr McCarus' points:

(1)  A 45-year-old with a history of normal Pap smears – risk is nil of cervical cancer.
(2)  There is a 50% increase of urinary incontinence after hysterectomy (*Lancet* 2000; **356(9229)**: 535–39.
(3)  There may be a role of pleasure during coitus if the cervix is retained, according to Masters and Johnson (1996), but this is questionable.

### *Advantages of LSH*

(1)  Decreased abdominal hematoma
(2)  Decreased estimated blood loss
(3)  Shorter Operating Room time compared with other laparoscopic hysterectomies
(4)  Faster discharge of patient from hospital
(5)  Faster recovery time and faster return to coitus (no vaginal incision).

### *Disadvantages of LSH*

(1)  4% chance of developing cervical stump cancer (continue Pap tests)
(2)  7% chance of cervical stump bleeding.

## Contraindications to LSH

(1) Cervical cancer
(2) Endometrial cancer
(3) Involvement of endometriosis of the cervix
(4) Abnormal Pap smears/dysplasia of cervix
(5) Cervical myoma
(6) Cervical prolapse.

---

**Pearls**

- During the informed consent process, one must include the possibility that if recurrent bleeding, spotting, or staining occurs – trachelectomy might need to be performed.
- The round ligaments have a dual blood supply (from the aorta and uterine arteries); therefore, suspect increased bleeding and use care in transection of these structures.
- The cervix is approximately 4 cm long – leave approximately 2 cm intact. In using the Harmonic ACE, coagulate approximately 4 seconds on minimal.
- For an LSH, essentially perform a REVERSE conization, leaving the uterosacrals and cardinals.
- Stay medial to uterine arteries until arriving at the uterosacral ligaments; then, begin the reverse cone, staying medial to the uterosacrals and thus taking the ascending vessels.
- Always sample the endometrium preoperatively, because MORCELLATOR will be used.

---

**Specific needs**

(1) Three trocars (one 5 mm and two 11 mm)
(2) Harmonic 5 mm ACE
(3) Laparoscopic uterine manipulator (*not* cervical manipulator)
(4) Self-righting needle holder (SRNH) and German needle holder (GRH)
(5) Morcellator
(6) Adhesion prevention (INTERCEDE, PRECLUDE, etc.).

---

**Technique**

After proper prep, drape, and placement of trocars – approximately 2.5 liters of $CO_2$ gas was insufflated into the abdomen. Round ligaments were grasped with the Harmonic ACE and coagulated for approximately 4 seconds on minimal setting and transected at 90° angles. Using strong traction with the uterine manipulator, the broad ligaments were transected using the Harmonic ACE. The bladder was dissected using laparoscopic scissors and Endo Peanuts.

The uterine vessels were carefully placed on traction using the uterine manipulator. The Harmonic ACE was then placed at a 90° angle and held motionless as a 4-second coagulation and transection was performed on minimum setting. This was performed bilaterally.

Being careful to stay medially and using the Harmonic ACE, consecutive drilling, clamping, and maximum settings were performed to take the lower uterine segment from the cervix. Continued use of the Harmonic ACE, making certain that strong traction was used with the uterine manipulator and staying medially, the reverse cone was performed until meeting in the middle. The uterine corpus and much of the lower uterine segment was dropped to the side while the active blade of the Harmonic ACE was placed into the cervical canal, and this was coagulated for 20 seconds using minimum settings on the ACE. *(The cervical stump may be reapproximated with deep bites using the SRNH, GRH, and 3-0 Monocryl. INTERCEDE can be placed through one of the laparoscopic ports and placed on top of the sutured cervix or over an unsutured cervix if hemostasis is excellent.)*

Eventually, the morcellator was placed through the 11 mm incision without port. The uterine tissue was pulled up into the morcellator and fed into the blade until there was no more uterine tissue visualized in the abdomen.

Laparoscopic irrigation was performed and hemostasis was judged to be excellent. All instruments were removed via laparoscopic visualization. Hemostasis was again considered excellent at all port sites. Incisions were closed with _____ (0 Vicryl) along the fascia and _____ (5-0 Vicryl) along the skin in subcutaneous fashion. Band-Aids were applied over the cleansed incisions. All needle, instrument, and sponge counts were correct. The patient went to the PACU in excellent condition.

## MINIMALLY INVASIVE VAGINAL HYSTERECTOMY

MIVH was first developed and the term coined by the author several years ago. A better way to avoid ANY abdominal incisions and accomplish the TVH in a more minimally invasive and quicker manner to afford the patient the fastest and best recovery for hysterectomy was the goal. MIVH is the best way to perform a hysterectomy if at all possible.

Common excuses for not performing an MIVH include previous C-section or surgeries, potential adhesions, large size of the uterus, pathology, ovaries/tubes need removal, small introitus, immobility of the uterus, and small pelvis. However, the author has shown that the above excuses are only excuses and that, regardless of these pre-op factors, after thousands of MIVHs with the above pre-op factors, successful MIVH was performed without significant complications.

### Advantages of MIVH

(1)  Less pain than ANY other hysterectomy
(2)  Faster recovery than ANY other hysterectomy
(3)  Quickest return to normal activity
(4)  Least amount of bowel manipulation
(5)  Least compromise to pulmonary system
(6)  Avoids ANY incisional complication
(7)  Increases ambulation
(8)  Least amount of PONV than ANY other hysterectomy
(9)  Allows correction of vaginal relaxation at same time
(10)  No shoulder pain or bloating due to $CO_2$ gas retention
(11)  No concern for abdominal herniation
(12)  Cosmetic
(13)  Reduced instrumentation requirements
(14)  Overall reduced procedure cost
(15)  Reduced operative time versus abdominal- or any laparoscopic-type hysterectomy. In fact, according to a 2002 study in the *Journal of Pelvic Surgery*, Kovac and Thompson showed that the use of the endocutter significantly reduced overall operative time for even vaginal hysterectomy from 49 minutes (TVH) to 34 minutes (MIVH).

### Disadvantages of MIVH

(1)  Requires additional training and preceptoring
(2)  Requires knowledge of the pelvic anatomy and enough cases to feel comfortable with the 'feeling' of less visualization and manipulation.

### Specific needs

(1)  Odansetron 8 mg ODT (orally disintegrating tablet) pre-op and post-op
(2)  Broad-spectrum antibiotic pre-op
(3)  Marcaine (bupivacaine) with 0.5% epinephrine
(4)  Bovie with 90° tip
(5)  Auvard (shortbill) and Steiner-Auvard (duckbill) weighted retractors
(6)  Ethicon ETS Flex45 Articulating Endoscopic Linear Cutter with at least 4–6 white or blue reloads. (During Dr Turrentine's study and experience with the development and teaching MIVH, many options were tried, including LigaSure and other devices, but the Ethicon ETS Flex45 had the least amount of complications)
(7)  JET pack (McNeil #40120)
(8)  Dental mirror with alcohol in sterile cup or other anti-fog material.

**Pearls**

- Know your staples:
  Gray – 0.85 mm closed staple height (6 row)
  White – 1.0 mm closed staple height (6 row)
  Blue – 1.5 mm closed staple height (4 or 6 row)
  Green – 2.0 mm closed staple height (4 row).
  Grays are usually only used on mesentery. These have been used in over 60 vaginal appendectomies along the mesoappendix. White and/or blue are most often used during the procedure, depending on the thickness of the tissue. Green reloads are rarely used, except on extremely thick tissue.
- Blood loss should be minimal. Most patients leave within 2 hours after an MIVH. However, if a post-op hematocrit should drop more than 3%, the patient should be placed on further observation, possibly until the next morning.

**Technique**

The patient was placed in the candy cane stirrups and appropriate adjustments were made to avoid injury to nerves or other structures of the legs. Hips were adjusted at the edge of the table. The patient was prepped and draped in a routine manner using _____ (Betadine or Hibiclens). The bladder was emptied by catheter and the catheter removed. An Auvard-weighted speculum was placed in the vagina. The anterior and posterior lip of the cervix was grasped with a thyroid (Lahey) clamp and retracted appropriately to enable the injection of 0.5% Marcaine (bupivacaine) with epinephrine.

A Bovie, with settings 70/50 to cut and coagulate with 90° angled tip, was then used to create anterior and posterior incisions of the cervicovaginal junction. The vagina was then sharply and bluntly dissected with Mayo scissors and single strung-out sponge. Once the 'white line' of the vesicoperitoneal fold was identified and cut, the anterior cul-de-sac was identified by the observation of yellow fat. A right-angle retractor was placed here. The posterior cul-de-sac was then entered sharply. Peritoneal reflection was noted and the Auvard retractor was replaced with a Steiner-Auvard retractor.

Z-clamps were placed on the cardinal/uterosacral ligaments bilaterally, cut with Mayo scissors, and ligated with _____ (0 Vicryl) suture, leaving a long tag on both sides and tagged with hemostats. Using the Ethicon ETS Flex45 stapling/cutting device along the uterine vessels and broad ligaments bilaterally, the uterus became much more mobile. With the aid of some moderate Trendelenburg position and the use of a damp 'JET' pack that was placed into the posterior cul-de-sac, visualization was excellent and other structures were pushed away from harm.

The Ethicon ETS Flex45 was then activated on the utero-ovarian and round ligaments *(may be used on the infundibulopelvic ligaments if adnexa are to be removed per BSO)* and the uterus was easily removed.

The peritoneum was examined with dental mirrors, with close attention to the pelvic side-walls. The peritoneum was then closed, removing the JET pack simultaneously, as a purse-string stitch (using a long 0 Vicryl suture) was ligated, making certain to incorporate the broad, uterosacral, and cardinal ligament stumps. *(Closing the peritoneum can actually be skipped after dental mirror inspection and removal of JET pack if necessary due to the next step.)* The tagged Vicryl sutures that contained the cardinal/uterosacral complex were then used to close the pelvic floor. This area was liberally irrigated and then the vaginal cuff was closed with several sutures. Hemostasis was excellent. Sponge, lap, instrument, and needle counts were all correct. The patient's bladder was emptied again with a catheter and her legs were removed from the stirrups. She went to the PACU in excellent condition.

# Hysteroscopy

**Important points**

*Contraindications to hysteroscopy*

IUP, PID, invasive endometrial cancer.

*Distending media*

Drawbacks:

## $CO_2$

(1) Hypercarbia
(2) Acidosis
(3) Cardiac arrhythmias
(4) Cardiac arrest
(5) Embolization
(6) Death.

## D5W

(1) Low viscosity
(2) Low ability to disperse blood from field

## 32% Dextran 70 (Hyskon)

(1) Excessive fluid absorption . . .

    (a) hyponatremia
    (b) pulmonary edema
    (c) DIC and coagulation defects
    (d) anaphylactic reactions

(2) Adherence to instruments can damage valves and optical components
(3) Care must be taken not to overdilate the cervix or Hyskon will drain too quickly and make distention difficult.

## Mannitol 5% or 3% solution

(1) Hypervolemia with acute pulmonary edema (especially in renal compromised patients)
(2) Can also cause osmotic diuresis and subsequent hypovolemia.

### Sorbitol 3% or 3.3% water solutions

Less likely to cause water intoxication as others, but can cause hyperglycemia.

### Cytal 3% solution (combination of sorbitol 2.7% and mannitol 0.54%)

(1) Very expensive
(2) Increased risk for bacterial contamination.

### Glycine

(1) Although it is less likely to cause water intoxication, glycine can cause temporary blindness
(2) It may cause seizures or encephalopathy by enhancing the effects of *N*-methyl-D-aspartate (NMDA), an excitatory neurotransmitter, and by increasing the absorption of ammonia
(3) Ammonia toxicity (prophylactic IV administration of arginine can blunt the increase in serum ammonia concentration when the use of media containing glycine is planned)
(4) Hyperoxaluria has also been described.

---

**Pearls**

- Hysteroscopic myomectomy is the hysteroscopic procedure most frequently associated with water intoxication syndrome.
- Never use a laparoscopic insufflator to insufflate or distend the uterine cavity. (Hysteroflator automatically shuts off at 200 mmHg.)
- Glycine-associated seizures are initially treated with IV magnesium. The mechanism of water intoxication syndrome involves decrease in serum sodium concentrations.
- The average fluid absorption during hysteroscopic myomectomy is 20 ml/min.
- Patients undergoing hysteroscopy are at risk for hypothermia.
- Plasma sodium deficit should be corrected at a rate of 1.5 mEq/h.
- Limiting resection time to less than 1 hour may decrease the risk of developing water intoxication syndrome.

---

## HYSTEROSCOPIC ABLATION OF THE ENDOMETRIUM

---

**Author's notes**

Following transcription for diagnostic hysteroscopy that proceeded a comment in regards to preoperative therapy such as danazol 600–800 mg daily for 4 weeks or Synarel (nafarelin) 7.5 mg, Lupron (leuprolide), etc . . ., to produce atrophic and thin endometrium, the following transcription can be applied.

---

**Technique**

_____ (6–8 ml) of a dilute solution of vasopressin (10 units in 10 ml sterile saline) was injected into the cervical and paracervical areas to decrease blood loss. Dilation of the cervix to _____ (9–10 mm) was performed to accommodate the operative sheath of the 26F resectoscope. This allowed a watertight seal but with the ability to insert and withdraw the instrument. (Rollerball, rollerbarrel, or Nd-YAG laser can be used at this point but since rollerball and loop electrode is the author's preference, this is transcribed.)

Uterine distention was provided by a _____ (3% sorbitol, glycine, etc.) solution fed into the inflow port on the sheath and collected by low suction from the outflow port. Cutting current of _____ (usually 120 W) and a coagulation current of _____ (65 W) were utilized as major _____ (lesions, myoma, etc.) were shaved with the resectoscope loop electrode to the level of the endometrium. Care was taken to avoid perforation of the myometrium. The rollerball electrode was used along the cornu and lower uterine segment, using combination resection and coagulation to a depth of _____ (3–4 mm). The loop and rollerball were used interchangeably until the result was noted to be (good, excellent, describe).

The procedure was then discontinued and instrumentation removed from the pelvis. The patient tolerated the procedure very well.

## Alternative endometrial ablation techniques

### Example (HerOption)

Knowing that the patient had sufficient benign endometrial sampling results, the patient underwent HerOption. Peracervical block was performed after routine prep and drape. Transabdominal ultrasound was performed and the uterus was sounded. The cryoprobe was placed at the fundus and angled toward the patient's right uterine cornu. The probe was visualized by ultrasound. The MINUS button was pushed to initiate the freeze. The CryoZone was monitored on ultrasound. At the appropriate time of _____ (6–9 minutes), the PLUS button was pushed to initiate warm. The probe was removed to the internal os and repositioned toward the contralateral side. It was made certain that the probe reached the second cornu. The MINUS button was pushed to initiate the freeze again. The CryoZone was monitored again on ultrasound. After the correct time was noted by computer, the PLUS button was pushed to warm the probe again. The procedure was discontinued at this time.

Some of these procedures can be performed in the office; others require anesthesia. Key facts for each are:

**HerOption** *endometrial cryoablation* (AMS Gynecology), 94% 4-year success rate, and uses a 5-mm diameter probe. Cryoanesthesia results in little pain for patient; IV sedation not required. Treatment time: 12–18 minutes. Depth of ablation: 9–12 mm. Ultrasound guidance provides individualized treatment and control of the depth of tissue destruction. Large uteri can be treated.

**Thermachoice**   *hot water balloon* (Gynecare), 89% 4-year success rate, and uses 5.5-mm diameter probe. Pain from heat and IUP. Treatment time: 8 minutes. Depth of ablation: 3–4 mm. Requires normal size and shape of uterus. Less likely to offer complete coverage of the endometrium.

**Hydro ThermAblator**   *free-flow hot water* (Boston Scientific), 91% 4-year success rate, and uses 8-mm diameter probe. Dilation and heat necessitate anesthesia; not appropriate for office use. Treatment time: 10 minutes heat; 17 minutes total. Depth of ablation: 2–4 mm. Hysteroscopically guided. There are reports of free-flow hot water resulting in vaginal burns. Large uteri can be treated.

**NovaSure**   *bipolar mesh* (NovaCept), 91% 3-year success rate, and uses an 8-mm diameter probe. Dilation, heat, and suction require anesthesia for patient tolerance. Treatment time: 90 seconds energy time; 10 minutes total. Depth of ablation: 2–9 mm. No pre-treatment recommended. Requires normal shape and size of uterus.

**MEA**   *microwave wand* (Microsulis), 83% overall satisfaction rate at 5 years, and uses a 9-mm diameter probe. Dilation requires anesthesia. Treatment time: 5–7 minutes. FDA approval? Most studied of these therapies (>2000 cases reported in European studies).

## HYSTEROSCOPIC BALLOON TUBOPLASTY (TRANSVAGINAL FALLOPIAN TUBE RECANALIZATION)

### Technique

After proximal tubal obstruction had been demonstrated by hystero-salpinography (HSG) and the patient had been given 2 days of prophylactic oral antibiotics consisting of _____ (doxycycline or Augmentin), the patient's follicular phase of her menstrual cycle was confirmed prior to beginning the procedure.

The patient was given IV _____ (Fentanyl or Versed), as needed, while her vital signs were monitored by _____ (Dynamap, nurse's name, etc., . . . ). The cervix was prepped with _____ (Betadine, Hibiclens) after bivalve speculum was in proper position.

The cervix was then cannulated by means of a coaxial angiographic catheter and guide wire system consisting of a _____ (6F) catheter and a (0.038 inch J-wire) The catheter was advanced to the ostium of the occluded tube and wedged into the ostium. Hyskon (or other radiographic material) was injected but did not clear the tubal obstruction. *(In some cases this clears the obstruction.)*

A smaller _____ (3F) catheter with a smaller, flexible _____ (0.018 inch) guide wire was advanced in a bougie type of dilatation through the interstitial portion of the fallopian tube until recanalization could be confirmed with _____ (Hyskon or other contrast material) being noted to demonstrate a fully patent fallopian tube.

The procedure was repeated with the opposite fallopian tube, as above, until patency was confirmed.

## DIAGNOSTIC HYSTEROSCOPY

### Technique

Bimanual examination was performed to determine the size of the uterus and the orientation of the corpus in relation to the cervix. Vaginal preparation was performed using _____ (Betadine, Hibiclens), then further disinfection was performed over a wide area of the exposed cervix after the _____ (bivalve, weighted, and Simons) speculum provided good exposure.

Distending media using _____ ($CO_2$, glycine, D5W, 32% Dextran 70, see above) was set at a flow rate not to exceed _____ . A single-toothed tenaculum was placed on the anterior cervical lip and held with the left hand. Traction corrected for _____ (anti, retro) version. Optical assembly and end of the hysteroscope was inserted into the external cervical os. The endocervical canal was examined and found to _____ (be within normal limits or describe pathology). The plicae palmatae was readily visible.

Instrumentation was advanced until resistance was met, then after _____ (10–20 seconds) the _____ (distention media) dilated the internal os enough to allow further advancement into the uterine cavity under _____ (direct, video) visualization. The flow rate was then maintained at _____ (ml/min) to allow systematic examination of the anterior, posterior, side-walls, fundus, and cornua of the intrauterine cavity. (Describe findings.)

## HYSTEROSCOPIC MYOMECTOMY

### Author's notes

Assuming the patient wishes to maintain fertility, this procedure is transcribed in the following manner. Otherwise, laser ablation or cautery would be considered an option. After inspection of the uterus, describe the findings.

**Technique**

After distention of the uterus with _____ (D5W, sorbitol, glycine, or Dextran 70, etc.), inspection of the uterus was performed. The large pedunculated fibroid was excised by transecting its stalk with the hysteroscopic scissors and controlling minimal bleeding with the _____ (cautery or laser). A smaller pedunculated fibroid was twisted off and extracted with the hysteroscopic polyp forceps. The submucous components of the intramural fibroids that were less than 2 × 2 cm were resected by placing the resectoscopic loop behind the tumor and drawing it toward the endoscope while applying _____ (30–40) watts of cutting current. Care was taken to avoid the tubal orifices while the resectoscope was used to shave the tumor into slices. Measuring _____ (4 mm × 3 cm for example), these floated in the (sorbitol, Dextran 70, D5W, etc.). These shavings and fragments ran out, as the resectoscope was withdrawn from its sheath. The remainder of the tissue pieces were pulled out with the hysteroscopic ovum forceps. The uterus was irrigated with normal saline to remove clots, bubbles, and debris; then the resectoscope was reinserted, the uterus redistended, and the operation continued in a similar manner until all myomae were absent.

The patient tolerated the procedure very well. Instructions had been given to her that included two doses of prophylactic antibiotics consisting of _____ . She was also given a 10-day course of _____ (po estrogen, Premarin, Ogen, Estrace) in the dose of _____ (usually 1.25 mg daily). She was to avoid coitus for (3–4 weeks) and had been advised to undergo a hysterogram approximately _____ (2–3) months postoperatively.

**ESSURE**

After the patient was properly prepped and draped, the hysteroscope was advanced per routine. With the endometrium visualized and left cornu located, the Essure catheter was inserted through the vagina, uterus, and into the fallopian tube, where the small metal implant (Essure) was deposited. The same procedure was repeated on the right fallopian tube. The procedure was then discontinued as all instrumentation was removed from the vagina. The patient was advised to use alternate contraception for at least 3 months following insertion of the implants until proper implant placement is confirmed by HSG.

## HYSTEROSCOPY FOR UTERINE SEPTAL RESECTION

### Technique

After a dilute solution of _____ (sorbitol, Dextran 70, etc.) was provided through a _____ (9–10 mm) dilated cervix, the hysteroscopic scissors were used to cut central and lateral scars. *(Sometimes passing the scissors between the scope and the endocervical canal offers the greatest opportunity for free hand surgery. Transcribe whether the instrument is passed through the sheath or between the scope and endocervical canal.)* After all the adhesions had been lysed, tubal patency was checked via injection of methylene blue. Laparoscopically, the patency of the tubes appeared _____ (bilaterally adequate, only unilaterally to spill, etc.).

After tubal patency was evaluated, a _____ (Lippes loop) was inserted to help separate the uterine walls. The patient was then placed on _____ (high-dose estrogens, Premarin 1.25 mg po qid for two 21-day courses, separated by 1 week of rest). The patient tolerated the procedure well and has been instructed to have the IUD removed after the end of her two treatment periods and then undergo another HSG.

---

### Author's notes

Diagnostic hysteroscopy is done first if this is also performed in conjunction with laparoscopy, so perforation can be ruled out as a possible complication. Solos offers a dual camera system that is excellent for performing laparoscopy and hysteroscopy simultaneously.

If significant bleeding occurs, a Silastic rubber balloon can be used as a tamponade by inflating it for several hours, then reducing the pressure and leaving it in place for up to 1 week.

# Inguinal and groin node dissection

### Technique

The femoral canal was dissected in a manner that allowed the tissue to be removed from the surrounding artery and vein. Cloquet's nodes (nodes of Rosenmüller) were located at the femoral ring beneath the inguinal ligament. They were dissected with Metzenbaum scissors and sent for frozen section. *(If these are negative for any metastatic disease, the dissection for vulvar disease can be considered complete.)*

The deep inguinal chain was dissected by opening the inguinal canal from the external inguinal ring. The round ligament that passes into the canal from the peritoneal cavity (where the inguinal ring begins) was excised and the deep inguinal lymphatic tissue was removed.

The extraperitoneal pelvic lymphadenectomy was initiated by opening the external oblique muscle 2 cm above the inguinal ligament. The incision was extended as far laterally as necessary for exposure through the internal oblique and transversalis muscles. The iliac vessels were exposed by retracting the peritoneum medially.

The external iliac, common iliac, and upper portion of hypogastric vessels were included in the dissection as the entire obturator space was thoroughly cleaned. The inferior epigastric artery and vein were ligated with 2-0 _____ (silk) suture. This was performed at the point where these vessels originated from the external iliac vessels, just inside the inguinal ligament, as they coursed upward to supply the abdominal wall. The ureter was displaced medially with the parietal peritoneum so as to avoid injury during the dissection.

Following dissection of necessary nodes, a _____ (Jackson–Pratt) closed-suction drain was placed in the retroperitoneal space as separate stab wounds were made in the abdomen for adequate removal of fluid and blood.

The inguinal canal was obliterated by closing the oblique and transversalis muscles in two layers using a #1 _____ (delayed absorbable) suture in a 'vest-over-pants' closure. The inguinal incision was closed without tension with suture and the groin specimen was sent to Pathology.

**Author's notes**

If Cloquet's nodes are negative for any metastatic disease, the dissection for vulvar disease can be considered complete.

Transposition of the sartorius muscle is not described here as prophylactic antibiotics have essentially eliminated the need for this portion of the operation in regards to radical vulvectomy.

# Laparoscopy

**Overview**

Operative laparoscopy can include operative laparoscopy with hydrochromo-tubation, laser laparoscopy, video laser laparoscopy, and innumerable other laparoscopic procedures other than diagnostic laparoscopy. Over the past 10–15 years, with the development of many stapling devices and coagulation/cutting devices, much of the laser surgery that was seen in the 1970s and 1980s has fallen out of use. In the 1990s and first 6 years of the 21st century, the dangerous complications of laser became past history. Bowel burns, ureteral and vessel injuries, and other complications are becoming less frequent with the development of newer and safer instrumentation such as the Ethicon Harmonic ACE. Many vessels can be safely transected, even those of 5 mm diameter with very little lateral spread of heat. Many of these laparoscopic procedures can be performed with the Harmonic ACE.

Most laparoscopic procedures, however, begin with basic steps in preparation for the operative portion of the laparoscopy. It is sometimes during this initial preparation that complications can occur. These complications can include injury to the bladder, puncture of a major vessel possibly because a second trocar was not being visualized during placement, or unrecognized injury to bowel because placement of a Verres needle was not properly tested to check for stool. Many surgeons have begun to use the bladeless trocars to visualize the entry rather than the blind use of the Verres needle or other trocars.

There are certain points that might be considered important while performing and then transcribing the medicolegal document of operative laparoscopy. The following operations will begin with the basic diagnostic laparoscopy transcription, then will become more specific for each individual operative procedure (in order to decrease redundancy).

In all laparoscopic operations, stick to the basics and do not forget to transcribe them . . .

Whenever laparoscopy is employed, video endoscopy is utilized (if possible). This is certainly not required or recommended, but advantages are:

(1) it allows greater involvement by the Operating Room team
(2) it allows assistants to really 'help' or 'do more'
(3) teaching potential is improved
(4) educational tapes or photographs can be produced
(5) patient enlightenment
(6) it increases referrals for surgery
(7) it makes possible better medicolegal documentation.

Some institutions, however, are not equipped with video laparoscopy, therefore, for the purpose of this book transcription will be directed to 'direct' or 'video' visualization. Very few hospitals are without video equipment in modern laparoscopy. Once familiar with video equipment, the operator can usually perform the entire surgery by watching the video screen without ever having to bend or look through the scope. However, a beam splitter can be advantageous over a direct coupler for video, since the beam splitter allows the operator to view directly in the pelvis but still obtain a good view on the monitor. This is very helpful when first beginning advanced laparoscopic surgeries. It helps the operator gain that 3-D visualization necessary to perform laparoscopy. Many trainers are available to the beginning student, along with cadaver or animal labs. These should be utilized prior to beginning the surgeon's 'learning curve' on human subjects.

There are many other important points to remember in performing laparoscopic operations, including constant irrigation fluid and/or smoke, being familiar with the equipment, and achieving adequate experience to be able to accomplish good results without too many complications. It is imperative, however, during and after this 'learning curve' that these possible complications be recognized if at all possible. It is also possible to reduce the number of complications if certain procedures are routine. This is another purpose of this book – to drill some of these 'routine' procedures into a 'form' transcription that one can read, perform, and transcribe over and over until these procedures are automatic.

---

**Important points/pearls**

- If a D & C is performed in conjunction with a laparoscopy – remember to be cautious for false passage ways and postmenopausal or postpartum (boggy) uteri that perforate easily.
- Always empty the bladder with a catheter prior to placing the Verres needle or trocar to decrease chances of inadvertent entry into the urinary bladder.
- Describe the type of trocars used such as disposable, sleeve retractable (Surgiport), bladeless, long, etc. . . .
- Describe the method or methods to test the placement of the initial needle puncture. Methods include:

  (a) 'Hanging drop method' – place one drop on hub of Verres needle and if it disappears down the needle, it indicates negative intra-abdominal cavity pressure.
  (b) 'Syringe method' – should indicate no resistance upon pushing the plunger with a few ml of sterile water into the abdomen.
  (c) 'Bubble method' – upon pulling the plunger of the sterile water-filled syringe back, bubbles should be noted rather than urine, feces, or blood!

---

(d) 'Gas pressure gauge method' – the $CO_2$ insufflator should not be in the red area or at a more than normal increased pressure (as would be noted if bowel, subcutaneous tissue, or other structures were against the bevel of the needle).

(e) It is not necessary to use towel clips to lift the abdomen for insertion of any trocar.

(f) Insert the trocar at the proper angle! Vessels lie deep!

(g) Watch *carefully* through the eyepiece or on the video screen when inserting the laparoscope through the sleeve. Laparoscopes can puncture cecums, omentums, and other structures that a sleeve may be directly against. If the bowel is entered, leave the trocar in place until repaired to prevent spillage of stool.

(h) Identify any injuries and correct these at the time of surgery. If there are no injuries and hemostasis is excellent, transcribe these observations.

(i) Do not risk causing an ectopic pregnancy or endometriosis. If chromotubation is planned, recommend surgery between the sixth and tenth day of the patient's cycle (if at all possible). This will avoid pushing endometrium or egg backwards through the tubes.

- Beware of single puncture laparoscopic procedures – under normal operative conditions, a 5 mm instrument protruding 10 mm or more beyond the distal end of the laparoscope will obstruct 14.6% of the operator's visual field.

- Physicians performing laparoscopic procedures must be able to perform the same procedure using open surgery methods in case of emergency.

- Carefully screen patients for laparoscopic surgery. Patients who are significantly overweight or have had previous abdominal incisions are not good candidates for your initial procedures.

- Avoid inadequate insufflation of the patient's abdomen. This will result in collapse of the abdominal wall, increasing the risk of trocar injuries to the abdominal cavity.

- Avoid excessive insufflation of the patient's abdomen (above 20 mmHg). This can result in carbon dioxide embolus.

- Do not blindly insert the trocar. Trocars blindly inserted above the patient's midline can result in injury to the iliac or epigastric vessels. Instead, use the open technique to make the incision and insert the trocar with direct vision or visualize the insertion via video if available.

- Perform your first 10–20 procedures under the guidance and supervision of a physician who has already mastered laparoscopic techniques. (The majority of all laparoscopic accidents occur during a physician's first 10 procedures.)

- In procedures that last longer than 30 minutes, use prophylaxis (hose, compression stockings) to prevent pulmonary embolism. In high-risk cases, administer subcutaneous heparin during the procedure.
- Inform patients that laparoscopy, compared with open surgery, may pose additional risks, and explain those risks in appropriate detail. Also tell patients that switching to the open procedure is appropriate if technical problems occur during laparoscopy.
- Key to success of operative laparoscopy is proper placement of second, third, and sometimes fourth ancillary puncture sites, which should be anterior and to either side of the tissue of interest, avoiding obstruction of the surgeon's vision or at an angle of poor visibility.

## ADHESIOLYSIS (LAPAROSCOPIC LYSIS OF ADHESIONS)

### Technique

Aqua dissection was performed using the tip of the _____ (Nezhat irrigator, aqua dissector) placed against the adhesive interface. The pressurized fluid created a cleavage plane that was able to be extended with further increased fluid pressure and blunt dissection. (Describe whether bowel–adnexa, tube–ovary, adnexa, pelvic side-wall, etc. . . . are being elevated and separated from each other.)

Sharp dissection using _____ (5 or 3 mm) hooked scissors was performed to lyse adhesions that were present between the tube and ovary. Vasopressin (20 U in 50 ml of Ringer's lactate solution) was used to promote hemostasis.

Electro dissection was performed using a (an) _____ (Elmore's, needle electrode, or other standard electrosurgical unit) and 3 mm laparoscopy scalpel with a cutting current of _____ (50–80 W) to divide dense adhesions. Bipolar desiccation at _____ (25 W) was used to control arteriolar bleeding.

$CO_2$ laser vaporization was also used interchangeably with the electrosurgical equipment. Aqua dissection was utilized as a 'backstop' by injecting fluid behind the adhesions during the lyses procedure. _____ (14 W) of power was delivered to the tissue using a _____ (5 mm) operating channel in a _____ (40 W) superpulse mode with a _____ (1 mm) spot size. (*The harmonic scalpel, hook, or Harmonic ACE is an excellent substitute for the laser to lyse adhesions.*)

At the end of the procedure, hemostasis was confirmed with 'underwater' examination by filling the pelvis with Ringer's lactate solution and all structures were examined for bleeding. (If there is any bleeding –

describe and coagulate with microbipolar forceps.) Prior to closure of the peritoneum, 2000 ml of Ringer's lactate solution was left in the pelvis to separate the structures during the initial stages of reperitonealization.

---

**Author's notes**

Transcribe the usual laparoscopic procedure for placement of laparo-scopic instrumentation (this can be found in the transcription sample of diagnostic laparoscopy). Usually if adhesions are expected to be severe, a vertical intraumbilical incision is made so as to accommodate a 10 mm laparoscope that can be attached to a beam splitter and video. Two additional 5 mm punctures are carried out along the pubic hairline after each has been visualized during placement.

If suturing is required to evert tubal ostia, excise omentum, etc., a modified half-hitch knot is tied loosely, allowing the knot to slide to the area being sutured, either freely or with help from a 3 mm laparoscopic needle-holder positioned at the lower-quadrant puncture site. The tapered 1 cm straight needle through a 5 mm short, self-retaining, trap-less trocar sleeve is already inside the peritoneal cavity. #0 catgut or 4-0 polydioxanone have been used for this method. Endo-loops are preferred by some if free ties can be used.

---

## ADNEXAL TORSION (LAPAROSCOPIC MANAGEMENT)

**Technique**

- Conservative management technique A & B: two additional 5 mm second-puncture trocars were inserted in the suprapubic line under (direct or video) _____ visualization. The affected adnexa was untwisted gently with atraumatic laparoscopic forceps to avoid any additional adnexal damage.
- Management technique C: gangrenous _____ (right, left, or both) adnexa were noted and there was no recovery after untwisting and observation for 10 minutes.

**Author's notes**

Transcribe the usual laparoscopic procedure for placement of laparoscopic instrumentation (see diagnostic laparoscopy).

Group A adnexa demonstrate no ischemia or mild lesions with immediate and complete recovery.

Group B are tubes and/or ovaries that demonstrate dark red or black ischemia but with partial recovery approximately 10 minutes after the pedicles were untwisted. (Whichever findings are noted are described, but Group B lesions should undergo a second-look laparoscopy 6–8 weeks after the initial procedure to assess recovery.)

The majority of torsion cases were caused by ovarian and/or para-ovarian cysts. Some of the etiologies can be abnormal length of the utero-ovarian ligaments. The cyst can be managed according to descriptions in this book. (Laparoscopic ovariopexies can be performed, using Falope rings to shorten the utero-ovarian ligament if it is too long, such as described in similar manner to shortening of the round ligaments for laparoscopic uterine suspension.)

Adnexa are usually removed laparoscopically or by laparotomy in scenarios such as seen in group C . . . describe and transcribe treatment.

## APPENDECTOMY

**Technique**

The appendix was lifted into view of the video camera using the laparoscopic grasper. The mesoappendiceal vessels were skeletonized by blunt dissection and occluded with 9 mm titanium clips using the ENDO-Clip applier as was necessary. Once the appendix was free, it was measured in thickness and then, using the _____ (gray, white) indicator, the appropriately measured multi-fire ENDO GIA 30 was placed across the appendiceal base and fired. The appendix was then released by the grasper, and the multi-fire ENDO GIA 30 was removed and a 5 mm grasper was placed through the 12 mm trocar using a reducer plate to prevent the escape of $CO_2$. The appendix was then withdrawn totally intact through the 12 mm trocar without difficulty.

The appendiceal stump was inspected closely to insure hemostasis and was irrigated with an antibiotic solution consisting of _____ (2 g Mandol in 1000 ml normal saline).

*(If one uses the stapler and the appendix requires two staple fires to be removed, staple across the appendix first and then the mesoappendix. This will decrease the risk of bleeding and/or retraction of the appendiceal artery that runs close to the base of the appendix through the mesoappendix.)*

---

**Author's notes**

Transcribe the usual procedure for a diagnostic laparoscopy, except use a 12 mm Surgiport trocar rather than the customary 5 mm suprapubic port, along with right and/or left lower quadrant 5 mm trocars, approximately 10 cm from the midline at a level midway between the umbilicus and the symphysis pubis.

Use 5 mm ports if endo-loops and/or laparoscopic suturing is planned to ligate, cut, and bury the stump of the appendix. However, at this time, if stapling devices are planned, a larger port would be necessary.

Cautery and Roeder chromic loops can be used for hemostasis of mesoappendix. The loops may also be used to ligate the appendix prior to transection, but these methods are becoming much less necessary with the innovative multi-fire ENDO GIA 30, ENDO-Clips, and other stapling devices.

---

## BLADDER SUSPENSION OR BURCH PROCEDURE

*The Capio suture-capturing device is very helpful in these cases if sutures are utilized rather than staples. Some clinicians also prefer to avoid mesh or sling devices.*

Transcribe routine placement of 10 × 12 trocars and 5 mm trocars bilateral to epigastric arteries per routine diagnostic laparoscopy.

Laparoscopic endoshears were used to create a 5 cm incision approximately 2 cm above the symphysis pubis along the anterior peritoneum and into the retropubic space. Bipolar forceps were used at least 2–2.5 cm lateral to the urethra to maintain hemostasis.

Two 1.25 × 1–2 cm of Prolene mesh passed through the 10 × 12 trocar and an Ethicon endoscopic stapler was used to place a staple into the perivaginal fascia, as the assistant used the index and middle finger in the patient's vagina to lift the urethra–vesical junction to identify the area to place the mesh. Two staples were then placed through the mesh into the center of Cooper's ligament. The bladder neck was checked to make certain it was at 1 cm from the symphysis pubis. The mesh was trimmed and excess was removed through the trocar.

The same procedure was performed on the opposite side. The retropubic space was irrigated liberally with Ringer's lactate solution, bleeding points identified, and controlled with bipolar forceps.

Peritoneum was reapproximated with an Endopath endoscopic articulating stapler. Trocars were removed as the abdomen and pelvis were inspected. These areas were found to be free of any injury, bleeding, or complication. The punctures were reapproximated with fine 3-0 _____ suture.

## CYSTECTOMY

### Technique

The cystic capsule was incised with _____ (scissors, laser, or unipolar electrode). A plane was found between the ovarian capsule and the cyst wall. Using the two lower abdominal 5 mm ports, graspers were used to peel back the capsule and the cyst was then teased out of the ovary by traction and counter traction. (This can be accomplished with the cyst intact or after it has been drained.) The cyst was slowly stripped out of the ovary and, after it was completely removed, the base was coagulated with _____ (the laser or bipolar forcep). The cyst was then removed by twisting it to allow compression of the tissue and then withdrawn through the _____ (10, 11, or 12 mm) sleeve. Copious irrigation was then utilized throughout the ovary and pelvis. Hemostasis was excellent and there was no injury to any pelvic structures. (A larger cyst or dermoid may be removed with a sac or through a colpotomy.) Instrumentation was removed, incisions reapproximated with _____ (3-0 delayed or 4-0 delayed absorbable) suture, and Neosporin with _____ Band-Aids applied.

### Author's notes

Document in transcription the result of the serum Ca-125, the absence of internal or external papillations on pre-op ultrasound, and make certain that proper work-up/documentation was present preoperatively to indicate laparoscopic removal of cyst.

Transcribe routine method of laparoscopic placement of trocars, $CO_2$, and pelvic findings.

## DIAGNOSTIC LAPAROSCOPY

### Technique

The patient was prepped with _____ solution and draped in the lithotomy position with special attention to the area of the umbilicus and cervix. Weighted speculum was placed into the vagina so as to expose the cervix. A _____ tenaculum was placed into the cervix to enable the uterus to be manipulated. The weighted speculum was removed and the bladder was emptied with a _____ catheter. Gloves were then changed prior to abdominal incision.

A small subumbilical incision was performed and _____ (Surgiport) Verres needle was placed into the incision and checked by the syringe, the hanging drop, the bubble, and the gas pressure register methods. All methods indicated proper placement of the needle.

Pneumoperitoneum of approximately 3 liters of $CO_2$ was established; then the_____(3 mm, 5 mm, 10/11 mm or 12 mm trocar) was properly inserted into the abdomen. The sound of escaping gas confirmed proper location in the abdomen as the trocar was removed from the sleeve.

Fiberoptics (and video camera if available) were connected to the laparoscope and this was inserted through the sleeve under _____ (direct or video) laparoscopic visualization. Trendelenburg position was increased and approximately 1–1.5 liters more of $CO_2$ gas was allowed into the abdomen to displace the viscera so as to easily visualize the pelvic organs. (Describe the findings.)

The procedure was discontinued and the abdomen was inspected. Hemostasis was excellent. There was no apparent injury to any bladder, bowel, vessels, or other visceral structures. The $CO_2$ was released from the abdominal cavity. All instrumentation was removed from the abdomen. The subumbilical incision was reapproximated with a figure-of-eight suture utilizing 3-0 _____ suture. Neosporin and Band-Aid were applied to the incision. All instrumentation was removed from the vagina and the patient went to the Recovery Room in excellent condition.

## ECTOPIC PREGNANCY – AMPULLARY SUCTION AND IRRIGATION

**Author's notes**

Transcribe routine method of laparoscopic placement of trocars, $CO_2$, and pelvic findings.

**Technique**

After finding the ectopic pregnancy near the ampulla, the tube was stabilized with an atraumatic grasper through the 5 mm port. Atraumatic grasping forceps were pushed into the tube and prongs were opened to grasp the protruding ectopic. A small irrigating and smoke evacuating system was utilized to obtain residual trophoblastic tissue from the end of the tube. Hemostasis was _____ excellent. (Although bleeding rarely occurs, it may be controlled by microbipolar forceps coagulation.) Approximately _____ (500–1000 ml) of lactated Ringer's solution was placed in the pelvis for flotation, then $CO_2$ released from the abdomen after making certain of hemostasis and absence of injury. Instrumentation was removed, incisions reapproximated with _____ , and _____ (dressings, Neosporin, Band-Aids) applied.

## ECTOPIC PREGNANCY – CHEMOTHERAPY OF UNRUPTURED TUBAL PREGNANCY

### Author's notes

Transcribe routine method of laparoscopic placement of trocar and/or trocars and $CO_2$. Transcribe the pelvic findings and describe in which tube the ectopic pregnancy was found. Mention that the abdominal pregnancy is 4 cm or less and also make note of the human chorionic gonadotropin (HCG) level. It is also suggested to have sonographic evidence, especially if video equipment is not available.

### Technique

A dilute solution of _____ (vasopressin 20 U in 6 ml NS (normal saline) or Pitressin (vasopressin) 0.5–1.0 IV) was injected gently into the meso-salpinx through a _____ (21-gauge) injection needle. _____ (10 ml) of methotrexate solution was injected gently at _____ (five or six) points between the tubal wall and the conceptus. (The dose of methotrexate given at first is 25 mg and amounts then decreased gradually thereafter to the final dose of 5 mg. A 50 mg dose vial is used so that 4 ml of NS is mixed with 1 ml of the 50 mg dose vial. This is usually injected first. Then 4 more ml of NS are mixed with the remaining 1 ml of 50 mg dose vial for final injections. Doses of methotrexate can range from as small as 525 mg.)

After hemostasis was judged to be excellent, the procedure was discontinued. All instrumentation was removed from the abdomen after as much of the $CO_2$ was removed as possible. (3-0 chromic) suture on an _____ (M-04) needle was used to close the subumbilical and lower abdominal incisions. Vaginal instrumentation was then removed.

## ECTOPIC PREGNANCY – SALPINGECTOMY (SEGMENTAL RESECTION)

### Author's note

Usually if the fallopian tube is severely damaged or contains an ectopic pregnancy larger than 3 cm, removing the tube or portion of the tube may be easier, safer, and may provide better assurance of complete evacuation of the problem than salpingotomy. Future microsurgical anastomosis can restore potency if only segmental resection is done. Document the reasoning of performing salpingectomy, transcribe routine laparoscopic placement of $CO_2$ and trocars, and then the following.

**Technique**

The _____ (right or left) tube was free of bowel and other structures. (If the tube is adherent to the bowel or other structures, laparotomy is mandatory in most cases as the mesosalpinx has to be accessible.) With the 10 mm operating laparoscope and two lower operating trocar sheaths in place, the proximal portion of the tube was grasped with laparoscopic flat duckbilled bipolar forceps and then cauterized for approximately 10 seconds. The fallopian tube was then grasped again along the distal end of the affected area of the tube and again cauterized for approximately 10 seconds.

The laparoscopic scissors were placed through the operating sheath in place of the bipolar forceps and the cauterized portions of the tube were transected. The _____ (tube or tubal segment) was grasped with laparoscopic forceps through the 5 mm sheath and the bipolar forceps and scissors were used to alternately cauterize and cut the mesosalpinx beneath the affected tube.

The _____ (affected segment or tube) was then seized by one end with a forcep placed through the laparoscope's operating channel. It was then carefully removed with the laparoscope through the sheath. (The tube or tubal segment may need to be divided into fragments if it is so large as to prevent passage of the tube through the 10 mm sheath.)

There was no injury to the pelvis, hemostasis was excellent, and $CO_2$ was released from the abdominal cavity as all instrumentation was removed from the abdomen. The incisions were reapproximated with _____ (3-0 delayed absorbable) suture. _____ (Neosporin) and Band-Aids were placed over the incisional sites. Vaginal instrumentation was removed and the patient went to the Recovery Room in good condition. (Overnight observation may sometimes be considered to rule out intraperitoneal bleeding.)

## ECTOPIC PREGNANCY – SALPINGOTOMY (FOR REMOVAL OF ECTOPIC PREGNANCY)

**Author's notes**

Transcribe routine method of laparoscopic placement of trocars, $CO_2$, and pelvic findings.

**Technique**

After placement of additional lower abdominal trocars in the midline and near the hairline lateral to the inferior epigastric artery, the tube was stabilized with an atraumatic grasper. The mesosalpinx was injected with a vasopressin (20 U/100 ml) solution. This was accomplished by placing a long spinal needle directly through the skin of the abdomen and into the mesosalpinx, taking care to avoid blood vessels. Approximately _____ (10 ml) was injected. The fallopian tube was then incised directly over the ectopic bulge along the antimesenteric border. The incision was performed with a _____ (unipolar electrode needle or knife, or with a laser). After a short time, the conceptus began to extrude through the opening of the tube. The remainder was _____ (irrigated out using a Nezhat hydrosurgical irrigator or teased out with small grasping forceps) through the 5 mm port. The tissue was then removed through the _____ (10/12 mm) midline port using a _____ (spoon forcep or endopouch).

The tube and pelvis were then thoroughly irrigated with copious amounts of sterile _____ (fluid) until clear. The salpingotomy incision was left open. Hemostasis was _____ (excellent, etc., . . .). (If there is any bleeding along the tube, one suture of PDS, 4-0 Vicryl, or a small bipolar coagulator may be used to bring about hemostasis.) The laparoscopy was completed, no injury to any structures were found, $CO_2$ was released, instrumentation removed under _____ (direct or video) laparoscopic vision, and the incisions were reapproximated and dressed appropriately.

Serial quantitative beta-HCG level was drawn in the Recovery Room and the patient was given instructions to return weekly for repeat levels until persistent trophoblastic disease or pregnancy is ruled out.

## FULGURATION OF ENDOMETRIOSIS

### Overview

Endometriosis may be treated by many methods, including excision, unipolar or bipolar electrocoagulation, laser vaporization, hormonal therapy, thermocoagulation, and, for larger lesions such as endometrioma, either removal or opening and draining of the lesions with minimal intracavitary manipulation except washing. Thermocoagulation or laser therapy will be used here only because of the author's preference, need for brevity, and the belief that these modalities are probably safer than electrocautery because the area of destruction around the coagulation point is smaller than unipolar or bipolar electrocoagulation. When lasers are mentioned, $CO_2$ or Nd:YAG (with sapphire tip) lasers are preferred because of their depths of penetration, yet the depth of lateral damage is held at a minimum of around 400–800 μm. A sample finding for this particular transcription will be included so as to demonstrate various examples of endometriosis treatment. An even newer option for fulguration of endometriosis is the Harmonic ACE.

**Technique**

An endometrioma of the right ovary was noted measuring 3 cm in size. There were other nonspecific lesions that appeared to be endometriosis of the cul-de-sac and left ovary. The right ovary also appeared to be adhered to the uterosacral ligament and right pelvic side-wall.

Keeping the foot 'very light' on the _____ (laser, coagulator, or Harmonic ball) pedal, the right ovary was systematically lysed away from areas of the rectum and ureter, being very careful to avoid these structures. The _____ (Nezhat or other) suction irrigation probe was used to bluntly lyse these adhesions and thus lift up the ovary. An initial incision was carried out into the right ovary using the _____ (laser, Harmonic ball coagulator, Harmonic ACE, or other) on _____ (superpulse 3, spot size 0.5, fast mode, or minimal/maximum coagulation). The relaxing incision was then carried out in a circular fashion _____ (2–4 mm) around the initial incision. Using two sets of grasping forceps through the 5 mm ports, the lesion was then stripped away from the healthy ovarian tissue. This was then brought through the _____ (5 mm or 10/12 mm) port. Hemostasis was excellent. Irrigation was placed into the cavity using Ringer's lactate solution.

The 3 mm knife electrode was used to incise and drain areas of the left ovary with superficial endometriosis and deeper cysts suspicious for endometrioma. A cyst cavity was discovered in one area and this was irrigated with Ringer's lactate solution and then excised in the same manner as was performed on the _____ (right, opposite) ovary using 3 mm and 5 mm grasping forceps. The ovary fell back together naturally after removal of the cyst wall. The remainder of very small lesions, less than 1 cm, were fulgurated with a 3 mm _____ (point, hook) electrode.

Excision of several of the larger implants in the cul-de-sac were carried out using the _____ ($CO_2$) laser with a spot size of _____ and power density of _____ (as high as possible) to vaporize the margins of the lesion while preserving the lesion itself. These were removed through the _____ (5 mm, 10 mm, or 12 mm) port. The remainder of the lesions less than 2 mm were vaporized with the laser or coagulated with the _____ (point thermocoagulator or bipolar coagulator).

After the entire pelvis was inspected and found to have no other pathology indicative of endometriosis, hemostasis and absence of inadvertent injury was assured, and pneumoperitoneum was released from the abdomen. Abdominal instrumentation was removed under _____ (direct or video) visualization. Incisions were reapproximated using _____ (3-0 or 4-0 delayed absorbable) suture. _____ (Neosporin) and _____ (Band-Aids) were placed over the incisions. Vaginal instrumentation was removed. The patient went to the recovery room in excellent condition.

---

**Author's notes**

Transcribe the usual procedure for a diagnostic laparoscopy with the addition of 12 mm and bilateral lower 5 mm port placements if needed.

---

## HYSTERECTOMY (LAPAROSCOPIC-ASSISTED VAGINAL HYSTERECTOMY, TOTAL LAPAROSCOPIC HYSTERECTOMY, AND LAPAROSCOPIC SUPRACERVICAL HYSTERECTOMY)

See these operations in sections in the Hysterectomy chapter.

## MYOMECTOMY

Two sample transcriptions are presented here, as there are different circumstances of myoma.

---

**Technique I**

The myoma was grasped with a _____ ('double-toothed biopsy forceps' or, if the myoma is too large for forceps to hold, with a 'claw forceps'), through the 5 mm port. The stalk was then grasped with a crocodile forceps and carefully coagulated from all sides for approximately 30 seconds until hemostasis was thought to be assured. The myoma was then excised with laparoscopic hook scissors. Oozing was controlled with the _____ (point coagulator or laser). The myoma was then removed directly with the claw forceps through the 12 mm trocar sleeve. Thorough irrigation was then performed throughout the pelvis.

Hand-assisted discs are useful with large fibroids.

If the stalk is large in diameter, a Harmonic ACE is useful for cutting and coagulation. Frequently, the defect must be closed with laparoscopic suturing techniques and Interceed placed over the area to prevent adhesions.

---

---

**Author's note**

If necessary, morcellation and extraction or colpotomy can be performed for large myomata. The endo-morcellator is excellent for large fibroids but brisk bleeding should be expected throughout the procedure. It is imperative that the surgeon be trained and be competent in the use of the morcellator!

---

**Technique II**

After estimating the myoma's size and extent, 5 U of vasopressin in 100 ml of normal saline was injected into the base and capsule. Another 5–10 ml of the vasopressin was then carefully injected into the corner of each side of the uterus (to constrict the ascending branch of the uterine artery). Once the myoma was noted to be white due to ischemia, enucleation of the myoma was started.

The serosal capsule was endocoagulated with the point coagulator in a 4 mm wide band. The capsule was then incised with the laparoscopic _____ (hook, micro, or Harmonic ACE) scissors (or laser beam) to establish a cleavage plane.

The capsule was then systematically stripped off the myoma using the enucleator (heated to 120°C). The myoma was stabilized with a (myoma cork-screw or large claw forceps). Once the base was reached, care was taken not to lacerate the feeding vessels.

The myoma was then removed by placing _____ (an endo-loop, Roeder loop, or endoligature) around the base through the 5 mm port and securely ligating the feeding vessels so as to prevent retraction. The pedicle was then cut with hook scissors above the point of ligation. The myoma was detached by _____ (twisting or coagulating) the pedicle. The crater was then thoroughly irrigated with normal saline and inspected for hemostasis. The point coagulator was used as necessary. Interceed was then placed over the area. (If the crater was large) – an endosuture with a 3 mm needle holder was loaded into a suture applicator. The applicator was then fed through the lower abdominal 5 mm trocar. A 5 mm needle holder was then placed through the contralateral 5 mm port and used to pick up the needle, bring out to tie a slip knot, then pushed back into the pelvis with a push rod attached to the ligature to reapproximate the serosal capsule walls. Irrigation was again performed after suturing was completed using _____ (#) interrupted sutures of (4-0 to 6-0 PDS, etc.).

The myoma was then fed into the morcellator (or extracted through a posterior colpotomy or 12 mm port).

After assessing that hemostasis was excellent, and that no injury had occurred to other structures, pneumoperitoneum was released and instrumentation removed under _____ (direct or video) visualization. Reapproximation of the incisions with _____ suture, placement of Band-Aids, and removal of vaginal instrumentation completed the operation.

---

**Author's notes**

Embedded myoma cannot initially be grasped: this requires dissection of the capsule, then cork-screw placement for further dissection. The hand-assisted disc is also helpful in these cases.

If the base or pedicle is not considered very large and hemostasis is not of much concern, one may transcribe the following for removal: 'the myoma was detached by _____ (twisting or coagulating) the pedicle.'

If coagulation was performed, simply transcribe: 'hook scissors or Harmonic scalpel were then used to cut the pedicle.'

It is sometimes recommended to place a Robinson drain through a lower abdominal 5 mm port and into the cul-de-sac for approximately 24 hours following removal of the myoma or myomae.

## NEOSALPINGOTOMY (VIDEOLASER LAPAROSCOPIC NEOSALPINGOTOMY)

**Technique**

The patient was prepped with solution and draped in the lithotomy position with special attention to the area of the umbilicus and cervix. Weighted speculum was placed into the vagina so as to expose the cervix. A Hume tenaculum with cannula was placed into the cervix to enable the uterus to be manipulated and chromotubation to be performed. The weighted speculum was removed and the bladder was emptied with a _____ catheter. Adapter tubing with indigo carmine in a 60 ml syringe was attached to the cannula for injection of blue dye. Gloves were then changed prior to abdominal incision.

A small subumbilical incision was performed and _____ (Verres) needle was placed into the incision and checked by the syringe, the hanging drop, the bubble, and the gas pressure register methods. All methods indicated proper placement of the needle.

Pneumoperitoneum of approximately 3 liters of $CO_2$ was established; then _____ trocar was properly inserted into the abdomen. The sound of escaping gas confirmed proper location in the abdomen as the trocar was removed from the sleeve.

Fiberoptics (and video camera if available) were connected to the laparoscope and this was inserted through the sleeve under _____ (direct or video) laparoscopic visualization. Trendelenburg position was increased and approximately 1–1.5 liters more of $CO_2$ gas was allowed into the abdomen to displace the viscera so as to easily visualize the pelvic organs. (Describe the findings.) Chromotubation was performed to inspect tubal blockage.

After confirmation of the _____ (right, left, or bilateral) hydrosalpinx was made, a second puncture was carried out for the placement of the Nezhat smoke _____ evacuator and aqua-dissector. A third puncture was then carried out along the opposite lower abdominal quadrant for placement of an accessory forcep to be used for traction and tubal manipulation. Both second and third punctures of trocars and sleeves were performed under _____ (direct or video) visualization to insure against an unrecognized visceral injury.

The _____ ($CO_2$, argon, KTP) laser was set on _____ (usually high wattage of about 24–30 W with use of a superpulse mode). The laser was used initially over the thinnest portion of the distal tube, making an incision with the use of two grasping forceps for traction and counter traction. The tube immediately collapsed as the blue dye inside the tube flowed out. Radial cuts were then made along the tube using a backstop probe, being careful throughout the operation to avoid the thicker portion of the tube and stay clear of the mesenteric border where larger vessels were located.

After the radial incisions had been made, the tubal edges were everted outwards by setting the laser on 2–3 W in a defocused mode and firing the laser beam several cm from the lateral peritoneal edge of the distal tube. The results were like outward petals of a flower.

Copious irrigation with heparinized (5000 U/liter) Ringer's lactate was performed through the Nezhat irrigator over the entire flowered-back fallopian tube. Hemostasis was excellent. Chromotubation was then done and tuboscopy was performed with saline for tubal dilatation to evaluate the status of the endothelium of the ampullary portion of the tube. The amount of destruction was considered _____ (minimal, moderate, or severe). The patient's prognosis was considered _____ for pregnancy after the surgery.

The procedure was discontinued and the abdomen was inspected. Hemostasis was excellent. There was no apparent injury to any bladder, bowel, vessels, or other visceral structures. The $CO_2$ was released from the abdominal cavity. All instrumentation was removed from the abdomen. The subumbilical incision was reapproximated with a figure-of-eight suture, utilizing 3-0 _____ suture. Neosporin and Band-Aid were applied to the incision. All instrumentation was removed from the vagina and the patient went to the Recovery Room in excellent condition.

---

**Author's notes**

$CO_2$ laser can be used with this technique but it is easier to perform with the use of an argon or KTP laser – it is suggested that the type of laser be mentioned in the operative report.

---

## OOPHORECTOMY (LAPAROSCOPIC SALPINGO-OOPHORECTOMY — RIGHT, LEFT, OR BILATERAL)

**Technique**

The decision to possibly remove the _____ (right ovary and tube) had been made previously with the patient prior to the procedure. A 5 mm trocar was placed in the lower right abdominal quadrant and was visualized during the video laparoscopy. Another incision was made in the middle lower abdomen between the symphysis pubis and the umbilicus in order to place the 12 mm laparoscopic trocar. This was also visualized under video laparoscopy. Through the 5 mm trocar, a laparoscopic grasper was placed and the ovary was lifted into view with the grasper. Through the 12 mm sleeve a GIA 30 multi-fire unit was placed at the base of the ovary and fallopian tube along the utero-ovarian and infundibulopelvic ligament. The instrument was fired and released. Another GIA 30 multi-fire unit was then placed through the 12 mm sleeve and again placed at the base of the ligaments and fired. This allowed the fallopian tube and the ovary to be dislodged from their ligaments. *(Harmonic ACE can also be used to coagulate and transect the IP ligament.)*

A 5 mm adaptor to insure no escape of $CO_2$ was placed over the 12 mm trocar and a 5 mm laparoscopic grasper was placed through this and the ovary was grasped and pulled to the 12 mm trocar sleeve. The fallopian tube was able to be brought up into the 12 mm sleeve, but the ovary was unable to be pulled into the sleeve. Therefore, the sleeve was pulled up through the incision and once the sleeve was removed from the incision, the fallopian tube was in view of the skin. Using forceps, the fallopian tube and ovary were worked through the skin until the entire ovary and fallopian tube had been removed from the incision (see Author's note). *(To avoid using a 12 mm trocar, a 5 mm trocar can be used in its place. However, a morcellator might need to be used to remove the adnexa and one must have ruled out malignancy. The morcellator will still require an incision larger than 5 mm.)*

It was at this point that the procedure was discontinued and the abdomen was inspected while pulling the trocars out. Hemostasis was excellent and there was no apparent injury to any bladder, bowel, vessels, or visceral structures. The $CO_2$ was released from the abdominal cavity. All instrumentation was removed from the abdomen. The subumbilical incision was reapproximated with a figure-of-eight suture utilizing _____ (3-0 chromic) suture. The other two incisions were also reapproximated with _____ (3-0 chromic) suture. Neosporin and Band-Aids were applied over each incision. All instrumentation was removed from the vagina and the patient went to the Recovery Room in excellent condition.

---

**Author's notes**

Transcribe routine entry and operative report for diagnostic laparoscopy prior to other trocar placements.

A 5 mm trocar is placed in the lower right abdominal quadrant and *visualized during video laparoscopy* in order to insure proper placement and to insure there is no injury to abdominal viscera.

An alternate method to remove the ovary (see second paragraph) is to transcribe: 'The ovary was cut with laparoscopic scissors by holding the ovary up against the barrel of the 12 mm sleeve until the ovary had been elongated in order to slide up through the 12 mm sleeve.' A morcellator may also be used if necessary. An *endocatch* bag is often helpful to remove adnexa that are difficult to pull up through the 10, 11, or 12 mm sleeve. The use of the bag is mandatory if the adenexa is suspicious for malignancy.

It is sometimes necessary to place the 5 mm trocar in the lower abdominal quadrant opposite to the adnexa to be removed, according to the operator's preference.

---

## REMOVAL OF TUBO-OVARIAN ABSCESS (TOA)

### Overview

After presumptive diagnosis of TOA, arrange hospitalization for laparoscopy. The average rate of misdiagnosis of PID, as confirmed by laparoscopy, has been estimated as high as 35%. Even a seemingly obvious TOA may prove to be an endometrioma, hemorrhagic corpus luteum cyst, or abscess surrounding a ruptured appendix.

Reich described the role of laparoscopy in treating TOA and pelvic abscess in an Update on Surgery in Contemporary OB/GYN in 1989. He recommended that antibiotics be started usually 2–24 hours prior to laparoscopy. He recommended cefoxitin 2 g with oral doxycycline on postoperative day 1. Droegemueller recommends a regimen of clindamycin and gentamicin if abscess is suspected.

Reich offers that the advantages of laparoscopy over laparotomy includes less blood loss using the Aquapurator, less superficial and deep wound infection, dehiscence, bowel injury, bowel obstruction, persistent undrained pus collections, thrombophlebitis, pulmonary embolism, septic shock, and subdiaphragmatic abscess.

---

**Author's notes**

Transcribe routine technique for diagnostic laparoscopy combined with hysteroscopy during peritoneal insufflation to assess the endometrial cavity and take culture specimens. During the transcription of the laparoscopy and following the hysteroscopy, place a Cohen cannula in the endocervical canal for uterine manipulation and tubal lavage.

---

**Technique**

Second and third trocars were placed under _____ (direct or video) visualization just below the pubic hairline adjacent to the inferior epigastric vessels. A _____ (blunt probe or grasping forceps) was inserted through the right-sided trocar sleeve to be used for traction and retraction. A _____ (Nezhat irrigation/suction probe or Aquapurator) was inserted into the left-sided trocar sleeve. This was utilized to mobilize omentum, small bowel, rectosigmoid, and tubo-ovarian adhesions until entry into the abscess cavity. Purulent fluid was aspirated while returning the patient from 20° to 10° Trendelenburg position. Separate culture of fluid aspirate and inflammatory exudate were obtained and sent to Bacteriology.

The _____ (Aquapurator or Nezhat irrigator/suction device) was used to separate bowel and omentum from the uterus and adnexa. It was also used to lyse adhesions. The _____ (Nezhat or Aquapurator's) tip was placed against the adhesive interface between bowel, adnexa, and pelvic side-wall; thus the plane of dissection was extended bluntly using the tip and pressurized fluid stream. Grasping forceps were utilized to place tension on the distorted tissue plane for accurate identification. Necrotic inflammatory tissue and exudate of the abscess cavity was excised with a 5 mm biopsy forceps after dissection was complete. Irrigation of all cavities, holes, and fimbrial ostia was performed with the _____ (Aquapurator or Nezhat irrigator) to remove infected debris and lessen chances of recurrence. This irrigation was performed in a retrograde manner into the fimbrial ostia using grasping forceps to speed away the agglutinating fimbria. The fimbrial mucosa was assessed for its quality for future prognosis, which can be described as _____ .

Tubal lavage with indigo carmine through the Cohen cannula was attempted. Patency was _____ (absent or present). (Describe if any inspissated necrotic material was visualized being pushed through the tube.)

Liberal use of lavage was performed using Ringer's lactate until the effluent was clear. Approximately 1 liter of Ringer's lactate was flushed through the _____ (Aquapurator or Nezhat device) on each side of the falciform ligament in the upper abdomen to dilute any purulent material that may have entered these areas during the 20° Trendelenburg positioning. Reverse Trendelenburg position was then used to help suction as much fluid as possible away from the peritoneal cavity.

The laparoscope and irrigation/suction device was then manipulated into the deep cul-de-sac beneath floating bowel and omentum. Irrigation and suction was performed until the effluent was clear. Separation and hemostasis appeared complete.

Approximately 2 liters of fresh irrigant was left in the peritoneal cavity to prevent fibrin adherence between visual structures. There was no apparent injury to any bladder, bowel, vessels, or other visual structures. All instrumentation was removed from the abdomen.

The subumbilical adhesion was reapproximated with a figure-of-eight suture utilizing 3-0 _____ suture. Neosporin and Band-Aids were applied to the incision. The second and third puncture sites were approximated loosely with a _____ (Javid vascular clamp) to allow drainage of excess irrigant caused by possible intra-abdominal pressure. All instrumentation was then removed from the vagina. The patient went to the Recovery Room in _____ condition.

## UTERINE SUSPENSION

### Technique

The round ligaments were identified bilaterally. _____ (Two or more) Falope rings were applied on each round ligament, creating small loops. The round ligaments were noted to be shortened bilaterally, and the uterus was pulled forward. The round ligament appeared to be shortened by about _____ (3 cm).

There appeared to be no transection or bleeding. *(Dictate there is no bleeding if, of course, there is no bleeding.)*

---

**Author's notes**

Transcribe the routine laparoscopic surgery in regards to the evaluation of infertility or pelvic pain and placement of trocars. In a series of 150 patients reported on by Serour et al, transection and bleeding occurred in 3.33%.*

---

**References**

- Serour GI, Hefwani F. A new approach to the problem of retroverted uterus in infertile patients. Presented at the IXth World Congress of Obstetrics and Gynecology, Tokyo, October 25–31, 1979.
- Serour GI, Hefwani FI, Kandil O, et al. Laparoscopic ventrosuspension: a new technique. Int J Gynaecol Obstet 1982, 20: 129–31.

## UTEROSACRAL NERVE ABLATION (LUNA)

**Technique**

The uterosacral ligaments were placed on stretch by flexing the uterus upwards toward the anterior abdominal wall. The $CO_2$ laser, which was set at _____ (10–20 W/cm$^3$), was fired at the uterosacral ligaments at their insertions into the cervix. Vaporization was limited to the uterosacral ligaments using a back-and-forth motion of the laser beam. Bleeding was controlled by defocused beams while lasering was kept very superficial. *(Harmonic ball, hook, scalpel, or ACE can be used in place of the laser technique.)*

A superficial vaporization was continued in a U-shaped fashion across the base of the cervix to connect the two 'cut' areas.

---

**Author's notes**

Transcribe the usual laparoscopic procedure for placement of laparoscopic instrumentation.

Bleeding is controlled by defocused beams while lasering is kept very superficial. This is important to avoid further bleeding and/or injury to the ureter.

Any treatment of endometriosis, lysis of adhesions, or other surgery should now be completed and transcribed.

---

# Laser procedures

## MARSUPIALIZATION OF BARTHOLIN'S GLAND CYST

### Technique

After Betadine prep of the _____ (left or right) vulvar area and surrounding vulva and perineum, the colposcopic laser was adjusted to a power density of 900 W/cm$^2$ with a 1.5 mm spot size. Using superpulse 2, 0–2 seconds exposure rate, and moderate speed, a 1.5 cm oval neostoma was created, extending from the vulvar skin into the cystic cavity, following as closely as possible to the original duct tract. The 1.5 cm defect was created by moving the laser beam rapidly in a circular fashion, thereby vaporizing a cylinder of tissue from the vulva epithelium into the cystic space, resulting in the removal of the obstructed main duct. The cylinder of tissue removed was 1.5 cm in diameter. The beam of application was very precise in that the operating colposcope was used as a microscope by coupling this to the laser. A copious amount of _____ (dark reddish mucus, etc.) escaped upon entering the cystic cavity. A routine culture was obtained.

The gland was gently massaged until all free mucus had been expressed. The cystic cavity was irrigated with both sterile normal saline and Betadine, using Q-tips. The lining of the cyst was then inverted and sutured to the vaginal mucosa on both sides with interrupted figure-of-eight sutures of #4-0 _____ (absorbable material). Again, the area was thoroughly irrigated with Betadine and no drains or packs were left in place.

The patient has been instructed to refrain from intercourse for approximately 2 weeks and has been asked to return to the office in approximately 6 days for a follow-up. Oozing during the procedure was noted interoperatively but was easily controlled by decreasing the power density, beam defocusing, and using pulses. The tongue blade was also used as a backstop behind the Bartholin's gland to prevent any aberrant reflection of laser beam. The patient was found to be very hemostatic and a very good result was noted. She left the Recovery Room in good condition.

## VAPORIZATION OF CERVIX

### Technique

The metal bivalve speculum was inserted into the vagina, the cervix was exposed, and local anesthesia was placed in the cervix. The transformational zone and area of pathology were again identified by washing the cervix with a 3% solution of acetic acid. The smoke evacuating system and blood evacuating system were connected to the laser speculum. The laser was placed on a power density of 1800 W/cm$^2$. The power setting was placed on superpulse 3, with laser beam diameter calculated to be 0.5 mm, an exposure rate of 0.2 seconds, and with a fast mode of repeat delivery. The entire transformational zone, including the abnormal cytology and flat condyloma, were outlined with the laser beam. The outlined area was divided into four quadrants with short bursts of laser energy. This outline extended approximately 3–4 mm beyond the diseased area in the transformational zone.

Beginning at 6 o'clock position of the cervix, the laser beam was moved quickly over the tissue to be destroyed in the southwest quadrant. The southeast quadrant was then lasered in the same manner. The northeast and northwest quadrants were then lasered in similar manner. The laser beam was moved in multiple directions, including diagonally, horizontally, and vertically. Rapid movement of the beam was utilized. A minimum depth of at least 6 mm was achieved, with a 4 mm depth of normal tissue being obtained beyond the lesion and transformational zone. The defect was also lasered centrally, incorporating approximately 8–10 mm altitude.

Hemostasis was maintained with the same power density, utilizing a suction device to remove the blood from the operative site, and sometimes increasing the spot size to 2 mm for coagulation. The result was excellent, and the laser char was removed with swabs of 3% acetic acid solution.

The patient has been given routine postoperative instructions and recommendations, including recommendations for mild analgesic, instructions to refrain from intercourse, douching, and using tampons for approximately 3 weeks. She will return for postoperative check-up in 3 months for repeat cytology and possibly repeat colposcopic examination, if necessary.

## VAPORIZATION OF CONDYLOMA (RECTAL, VULVAR, CERVICAL, AND VAGINAL)

### Technique

The patient had been previously shaved of hair from the perineum and anal exterior and all external warts were vaporized along the perineum, posterior fourchette and neighboring skin was brushed.

An anal laser speculum was lubricated and placed into the anus. The blades were gently opened and the mucosa was inspected for any visible warts; these were vaporized utilizing low power densities of approximately 350 $W/cm^2$. The speculum was rotated clockwise to cover the entire anus. A wet sponge was placed above to seal the rectum and a vacuum hose was attached to the laser speculum to automatically effect the smoke evacuation.

When anal treatment was completed, a second speculum was placed into the vagina. The cervix was exposed and warty lesions were vaporized along the vagina. Using a long-handled spot size laser manipulator of 0.1 mm, the vaginal fornices were exposed and treated. The remaining vaginal walls were examined and treated. Microwarty changes noted on the vagina were also treated on the lateral vaginal walls and brushed by angulating the laser, and shooting between the blades of the speculum and the laser beam was reflected as necessary. The hymenal ring and vestibule were also treated.

The cervix was treated under 3% acetic acid solution, utilizing the same powered density to vaporize all surface flat condyloma. The procedure was then discontinued, all instrumentation was removed, and the patient was removed to the Recovery Room in good condition.

## VAPORIZATION OF VAGINAL INTRAEPITHELIAL NEOPLASIA (VAIN)

### Technique

The laser bivalve speculum and the posterior vaginal cuff were swabbed thoroughly with 5% acetic acid solution (white table vinegar). The cotton tip applicator was moistened with the 5% acetic acid solution and thoroughly swabbed throughout the posterior vaginal area. By withdrawing and rotating the speculum, the vaginal mucosa folded over several times, permitting an end-on view of the tissue. The lesions began to appear white and sharply bordered. A power density of 25 $W/cm^2$ and then 40 watts per $cm^2$ was selected and a spot size of 2 mm was utilized. Utilizing a spinal needle, 2% Xylocaine (lidocaine) solution was injected underneath the VAIN lesions and approximately 2 mm of depth was obtained during the laser vaporization to ensure complete vaporization.

After outlining each lesion and using the Iris hooks to obtain full vaporizing capacity along the border of normal tissue, the intraepithelial disease was removed using circumferential and cross-hatched methods down to the depth at which the lesion was initially found when the lesion was outlined.

Hemostasis was achieved by both defocusing the laser beam and also by using Monsel's solution. The lesions that were involved along the posterior vaginal cuff and hidden by folds were grasped with the Iris hook and averted so that the lesion could be treated. There was a lesion noted on the _____ (left middle third, for example) of the vagina and vaporization was performed as the tissue folded down over the end of the speculum blades, permitting end-on ablation of the lesion. Injection of anesthetic was necessary. There were some small warty lesions over the _____ (left or right third) of the vagina at the introitus and these were treated by passing the laser beam between the blades of the speculum; a small amount of bleeding was controlled by lowering the wattage and placing a small swab of Monsel's solution. After the therapy was completed, the 5% acetic acid solution was used again to inspect the entire vagina and there were no other lesions noted. The procedure was discontinued and the speculum was removed from the vagina. The patient went to the Recovery Room in good condition and has been given routine discharge instructions and recommendations.

# Laparotomy, exploratory

### Technique

The patient was prepped and draped _____ (in the routine fashion or as quickly as possible to obtain a sterile field). A (describe incision) incision was carried out along the skin. The subcutaneous fat was incised and fascia then entered. Fascial incision was extended with Mayo scissors. Rectus muscle sheaths were separated in the midline. Peritoneum was picked up with hemostats away from underlying structures. Care was taken while incising the peritoneum with Metzenbaum scissors. The peritoneal incision was then extended with the scissors.

Standing on the patient's right side, the right hand was placed into the upper abdomen. After appropriate washings were obtained (if this step is included), the right kidney, liver, gallbladder, pancreas, stomach, left kidney, and para-aortic lymph nodes were palpated in sequence.

### Author's notes

Findings are described and the remainder of the procedure transcribed.

# LEEP (conization)

**Technique**

Bivalve speculum was placed into the vagina and the cervix was swabbed with 4% acetic acid solution. Colposcopy had already been performed. Lugol's solution was placed over the cervix and the limits of the lesion were determined. A solution of 2% Xylocaine (lidocaine) with epinephrine (1 to 100 000) of approximately _____ (9) ml was mixed with 1 ml of sodium bicarbonate. This solution was then used to inject approximately 2 ml deep near the edge of the ATZ circumferentially and approximately 1 mm deep into the cervical stroma around the cervical canal for a depth of approximately 1 cm. The antenna plate was placed under the patient. A 2.5 cm electrode was attached to the sterile pencil unit and the current selector was placed on power _____ (#7) at 'blend filter-cut'. The tip of the loop electrode was moistened. The cervix was also noted to be moist. The loop was slowly moved in a vertical direction from _____ (6 o'clock to 12 o'clock) beyond the edge of the lesion, and with a steady slow motion, the loop was moved beneath the lesion and moved to an exit of _____ (12 o'clock) position without any drag. The excised specimen was removed and sent for pathological evaluation. Bleeding was minimal but it was necessary to use the ball electrode in the setting of coagulation current. Care was taken to avoid coagulating around the endocervical canal. Colposcopy revealed no further persistence of disease. The square electrode was then placed at the _____ (9 o'clock) position and moved to the _____ (3 o'clock) position at approximately 3–4 mm away from the canal and a plug of tissue was then removed from the canal. The 4% acetic acid solution was then placed along the crater with a moistened cotton tip applicator to further inspect for residual disease.

There were no further residual signs of disease. The canal appeared to be clear and smooth with a pinkish-orange epithelium. There was no evidence of any white-appearing or dense-appearing tissue. A ball electrode was used to further coagulate small bleeding points, and then a thick film of Monsel's paste was placed into the crater and held in place for approximately 45 seconds. At this point, hemostasis was judged to be excellent, and all vaginal instrumentation was removed from the vagina.

The patient tolerated the procedure well and went to the Recovery Room in good condition.

Preoperatively, the patient had been given postoperative instructions that included recommendations to refrain from coitus, douching, and tampons for approximately 3 weeks. She was also advised that a brownish-black vaginal discharge would be present for a few days to 2–3 weeks and that if bleeding or spotting persisted longer than 6 days that she should call the office. She will return to the office for a re-Pap in approximately 3 months.

# Marshall–Marchetti–Krantz procedure

## Technique

After the intra-abdominal procedure was performed and completed, semi-frog position under anesthesia and pelvic examination was performed. A #24 Foley catheter with a 5 ml bulb was inserted into the bladder and inflated.

The dissection into the space of Retzius was started after the gloves had been changed and sterile procedure was followed. Any oozing and bleeding that was encountered was controlled by pressure, individual ligature, and careful fulguration. The dissection into the space of Retzius was carried down toward the inferior aspect of the symphysis within 1 cm of the external urethral meatus. After inserting two fingers into the vagina to elevate the anterior vagina and bladder neck so that the sutures could be more easily and accurately placed, the catheter demonstrated the urethra and a balloon indicated the bladder neck and trigonal area. The sutures of #1 _____ (delayed absorbable) material were placed and consisted of two sutures on either side. Each suture was taken into the submucosa of the vaginal wall lateral to the urethra, into the fascia adjacent to the wall of the urethra, and then into the fibro-cartilage of the symphysis using a #4 Mayo round needle. During the placement of the suture, the curvature of the needle was followed very accurately to avoid breakage of the needle or laceration of the tissue. The assistant and myself then changed gloves and gown and the sutures were then tied and cut in pairs from below upward.

After adequate suspension, a suprapubic Silastic tube (#12F) was then inserted through the skin and into the bladder under direct vision for abdominal drainage prior to closure of the incision. Two small Penrose drains were placed on either side of the midline in the operative area so as to drain any residual venous bleeding that might occur following closure of the wound. Then, closure of the fascia and muscle along with the subcutaneous layer was performed in the routine fashion. Following the closure of the skin, a bandage was applied and the patient was removed to the Recovery Room in good condition.

# Marsupialization of Bartholin's duct cyst

### Technique

After routine prep and drape and under general anesthesia, a wedge-shaped vertical incision was made in the vagina mucosa over the center of the Bartholin's gland cyst following culture of the purulent material that was present. This was performed outside the hymenal ring. Incision was made as wide as possible to enhance the postoperative patency of the stoma.

The cyst wall was then opened and drained of its remaining contents and the lining of the cyst was inverted and sutured to the vaginal mucosa on both sides with interrupted sutures of #2 _____ (delayed absorbable) material. The area was then irrigated thoroughly with Betadine and there were no drains or packs left in place.

The patient was instructed prior to pre-op anesthesia that daily sitz baths should begin on the 3rd postoperative day. The patient will be seen in the office in approximately 2–4 weeks to evaluate possible secondary fibrosis or abscess formation. A Word catheter was considered but the patient disclosed no interest in having a catheter in place for 3–4 weeks. Therefore, marsupialization was performed. The patient left the Operating Room in good condition and is in the Recovery Room in good condition.

# Microscopic fallopian tube reanastomosis (cornual-isthmic anastomosis)

If the Ob/Gyn surgeon has not experienced operating with robotics, he should at least try it once. It is amazing the difference in precision that one achieves using this new technology. One can schedule a preceptorship through the Ethicon Endo-Surgery Institute in Cincinnati. This is an excellent procedure that can be accomplished with the da Vinci robot (since the suture is so small) and laparoscopic surgery can be performed with such precision in this manner. However, since most clinicians are not equipped with the robot due to the expense, the transcription sample will be given per microscope or loops. This also can be done with the regular microscope, but, for explanation purposes here, the following transcription will do.

The incision was made through the skin and down through the fascia. The peritoneum was entered with two hemostats and Metzenbaum scissors. (*Document the length of fallopian tube.*)

The microscope was adjusted to a magnification of approximately 10–20 times greater than normal so that a critical point could be reached in the anastomosis of the corneal-isthmic portions of the tube. Once the microscope had been adjusted to above the table and the patient had been placed in the supine position on an operating table, her legs were then placed in the Allen stirrups. The uterus was easily exposed because of vaginal packing that had been placed into the vagina prior to the procedure. Utilizing a continuous flow of Dextran 70 from a 500 ml bag at the head of the bed on an IV pole, the end of the IV tubing continued to control the flow of irrigation throughout the microscopic surgery. Methylene blue dye was utilized during the entire procedure through the Humi dilator so that it could be determined at which point the dye stopped in the fallopian tube. Utilizing microscopic fine straight vascular scissors, the fallopian tube was cut in an angle until the methylene blue was noted to be spilling from the approximate portion of the fallopian tube. A #2-0 nylon monofilament suture was threaded through the tubal lumen and placed within the uterine cavity. The same procedure was carried out through the luminal side of the distal segment. The proximal obstructed end was resected and the #2-0 nylon was passed through the oviduct and out through the fimbriated end and mesosalpinx was carefully approximated to eliminate any tension at the anastomotic site. Using a _____ (#8 or # 10) suture on a _____ (3-8 circle taper) needle, it was passed perpendicular to the surface of the oviductal tissue while elevating the edge of the tissue with left-handed forceps and simultaneously placing the needle through the tissue, avoiding any grasping of the tissue with the jaws of the forceps. Once the needle had been placed through the opposite lumen, being careful not to occlude muscularis or serosa, the suture was gently pulled with very short pulls and aligned with needle holes. This was performed to avoid damage to the tissue caused by angulation of the entry hole. The sutures were laid parallel to the oviduct and, with each suture taken, the fallopian tube was pulled closely to within the area of the cornua. Hemostasis was achieved using a high-frequency fine-needle cautery. The two-layer closure was performed using _____ (#8-0) suture. The patient was given _____ (Unasyn 3 g) IV intraoperatively. Irrigation was performed during the entire procedure and methylene blue was injected into the Humi dilator; it was noted that the left fallopian tube spilled dye. The procedure was continued in the same manner on the opposite side.

After the entire procedure was completed, the peritoneum was reapproximated with _____ (2-0) suture in a continuous manner using a nonreactive suture so that the chances of adhesive formation would be slim. Prior to closing the peritoneum, Interceed was placed over the entire operative area and between the fallopian tube and ovary. After the peritoneum was closed, muscle tissue was reapproximated with interrupted sutures of 2-0 (delayed absorbable) suture. The fascia was closed with 2-0 (delayed absorbable) suture and the subcuticular layer was closed with _____ (3-0 plain) suture. The skin was reapproximated with _____ (5-0 absorbable suture) in a subcuticular fashion and ¼ inch Steri-strips were placed over the incision with benzoin. The patient tolerated the procedure well. All instrumentation was removed from the vagina after proper dressing of the abdominal incision. The patient went to the Recovery Room in good condition.

# Myomectomy

This procedure can be performed laparoscopic, hand-assisted laparoscopic, or even using the da Vinci robot. However, for explanation purposes here, a simple myomectomy via laparotomy is described.

## Technique

The patient was prepped with _____ solution and draped in the standard fashion for a _____ (Pfannenstiel or vertical) incision. Surgery was continued through the subcuticular, fascial, muscle, and peritoneum with great care until the fibroid(s) was (were) located. A dilute solution of vasopressin 20 U in 60 ml of saline was injected into the cornual areas and into the lower uterine segment near each uterine artery. Approximately _____ (2–5 ml) of solution was injected into each area. Additional injections of approximately _____ (5 ml) were administered into the fibroid being excised as needed.

The incision was made into the pseudocapsule of the fibroid using a _____ _____ (Harmonic ACE, Harmonic scalpel, $CO_2$ laser, Nd:YAG laser with sapphire tip, or needle-tipped cutting cautery). The fibroid was then grasped with a towel clip. Blunt and sharp dissection were used to separate the tumor, leaving as much healthy myometrium as possible. The endometrium was avoided in its entirety.

The remaining stalk of the myoma was ligated with _____ (#2-0 delayed absorbable) suture and _____ (excised, twisted away). The crater was then irrigated thoroughly with Ringer's lactate. The 'dead space' was closed with _____ (interrupted or continuous) _____ (#2-0 polyglactin or #1 delayed absorbable) suture. The serosa was then closed with a continuous _____ (#4-0) baseball stitch, using a minimum of suture exposure, thus minimizing adhesion formation.

Copious amounts of irrigation using _____ (Dextran 70, Ringer's lactate, or Mandol/normal saline) solution in the amount of _____ (150 ml) was placed in the pelvis. (This can be left to act as a flotation barrier against adhesions or _____ .) The solution was removed from the pelvis and Interceed was placed over the operative surfaces. The peritoneum was then closed with a continuous suture of _____ (#0 delayed absorbable) suture. The fascia was closed with a continuous suture of _____ (#1 delayed absorbable suture). The subcutaneous layer was closed with _____ (3-0 plain) suture. The skin was closed with _____

(5-0 Vicryl) in a continuous subcuticular stick. The incision was wiped clean with a wet lap, dry lap, and then benzoin and Steri-strips were applied followed by a bandage. The patient's sponge, instrument, needle, and lap counts were correct. She went to the Recovery Room in good condition.

**Important point**

Avoid the use of vasopressin if the patient is hypertensive.

# Para-aortic node dissection

**Technique**

The posterior peritoneum was excised and opened with Metzenbaum scissors. The incision was extended to a level above the inferior mesenteric artery and vein. A narrow _____ retractor was placed beneath the upper peritoneal margin to expose the para-aortic and paracaval regions widely.

The dissection began along the lateral margin of the left common iliac artery and continued above the inferior mesenteric vessels. Each mesenteric base of each dissected node was clamped with a vascular clip. Care was taken to avoid injury to the lumbar arteries and veins that lie behind the aorta and vena cava. Extreme caution was used while retracting the vena cava during the paracervical node dissection so as to avoid injury to the vessel. The dissection was carried out along the lateral side of the right common iliac artery and extended on the side of the vena cava to the region above the inferior mesenteric vessels. The inferior and superior lymphatic vessels were clamped securely, excised, and ligated with _____ (#3-0 silk) tie on the tip of an _____ (Adson) clamp which provided excellent prophylaxis in preventing a subsequent lymphocyst.

*(If bleeding has been troublesome during the para-aortic node dissection, a retroperitoneal drain should be placed in the operative site and brought through the abdominal wall.)* The retroperitoneum was reapproximated with a continuous _____ (2-0 delayed absorbable) suture.

# Paravaginal repair

This procedure can also be performed laparoscopically by using the Capio suture-capturing device (Boston Scientific/Microinvasive, Natick, MA).

---

**Technique**

Following routine prep and drape, a Pfannenstiel incision was carried out through the skin. The incision was continued through the subcutaneous tissue and fascia so that the peritoneum could be freed from the undersurface of the rectus muscle but not entered. The recti muscles were retracted and the retropubic space was entered by incising the transversalis fascia at its attachment to the superior pubic ramus laterally until the obturator notch could be palpated while the bladder was drawn medially away from the sidewall of the pelvis. My left hand was inserted into the vagina while holding the bladder with a sponge stick. The lateral sulcus of the vagina was elevated and could be appreciated by notation of the prominent veins coursing down the lateral sulcus.

Key sutures were placed through the lateral sulcus beneath the prominent veins while elevating the lateral superior sulcus. Before releasing the needle, traction was placed on the needle holder, moving its tip toward the ischial spine. While palpating with the vaginal hand, this traction was carried backward until the external meatus of the urethra could be felt to be drawn immediately beneath the middle of the lower edge of the symphysis. The lateral pelvic wall bite was then carried out. This suture was tagged and not tied. Permanent _____ (3-0 Tycron) suture on a _____ (medium GI needle was used).

Following the key sutures that were made bilaterally, additional sutures were placed through the vaginal sulcus with its overlying pubocervical fascia and the pelvic sidewalls bilaterally. These sutures were placed at 1 cm intervals with continual interrupted placement dorsally until the last suture was placed at about 1 cm in front of the ischial spine. Once all the sutures had been placed, with the most ventral suture having been placed as close as possible to the pubic ramus, at least six throws were tied for knot security in each suture.

The retropubic space was irrigated with warm Ringer's lactate solution. Hemostasis was _____ (excellent, good, etc., . . . and if poor describe how it was corrected).

The fascia was closed with _____ suture. The subcutaneous tissue was closed with _____ . The skin was closed with _____ .

A bandage was placed over the incision. Estimated blood loss was _____ . Sponge, lap, instrument, and needle counts were correct.

# Pelvic organ prolapse and pelvic reconstruction

## Overview

The terms of pelvic organ prolapse (POP) have changed just like the surgery has changed over the past 10–20 years.

Cystoceles are now considered 'anterior defects'. If the defect is midline, an anterior repair might be appropriate. However, if lateral defects in the vagina are noted, then a paravaginal repair would be necessary. In fact, the cystocele can be caused by central, paravaginal, and/or apical fascial defects. Dr Cullen Richardson spent many hours at the Georgia Institute of Technology working with engineers there and discovered that (mostly) lateral defects are where the forces occur or either at the highest apical part of the vagina. Thus, lateral (paravaginal) defects are more common than midline defects. This concept changes the way we treat the 'anterior repair'. Traditional anterior repair (Kelly plication) was found to have a 50–70% failure rate. This was because surgeons were suturing poor tissue to poor tissue that would break again. There were 58% failure rates even when using grafts, and a 54% failure rate with 'ultralateral' repairs. So why still the high failure rate? There were obturator internus tears so if grafts were used and attached to the correct fascia there was improvement, but still a 41% failure rate was noted at 2 years after most anterior repairs if Vicryl suture was used. T Julian, in 1996, found that there were NO FAILURE RATES if *permanent suture* was used. There were some mesh erosions in his studies. Using grafts has improved anterior defect repair, especially with the new instrumentation that is available. For instance, the Capio suture-capturing device (Boston Scientific) can be used to attach the graft to the arcus tendineus fascia posteriorly. The graft should be cut into a trapezoid shape (approximately 8 cm apical, 6–8 cm in length, and 12 cm at the base).

A rectocele is considered a 'posterior defect'. The traditional repair included placation of the rectovaginal fascia. Anatomical failure rates were as high as 4–24%. Dyspareunia has been reported as high as 20–50% following posterior repairs. DEFECT-SPECIFIC REPAIRS must be the order of the present-day surgery for both anterior and posterior defects. Failure rates have been reported as high as 11%, even with defect-specific repairs; however, these have been lowered to almost none when permanent suture is utilized (2-0 Ethibond with a CT-2 needle is an excellent choice).

An enterocele is now referred to as an 'apical defect'. This might be due to a tear or 'split' of an anterior and posterior defect. If peritoneal fat is observed during surgery, there is an enterocele present!

Birth trauma is still considered the major culprit that causes POP, but C-sectioning every pregnant patient does not make a patient immune as many of us have all seen with the aging population of women that have never given vaginal birth but have POP.

Level I        Uterosacral-cardinal
Level II       Arcus tendineus ('white line')
Level III      Fusion of endopelvic membranes and perineum breaks.

The 'take home' message for performing pelvic reconstruction includes:

(1) Transvaginal defect-*specific* repair has advanced over traditional repair.
(2) Defect-specific repair should be used with grafts, given appropriate points are exposed.
(3) Permanent suture (Ethibond or Prolene) should be used in an interrupted fashion. Remember, Ethibond is braided so use liberal irrigation and pre-op antibiotics (Ancef).
(4) It is not necessary to close the peritoneum.

---

**Important points/pearls**

- Document evidence of uterovaginal prolapse or other indications (if present) if uterus is also removed at time of surgery.
- Document if injection of normal saline with or without vasopressors is used.
- Plicate the periurethral and paravesical fascia *carefully* and *firmly* so as to elevate the proximal urethra and urethrovesical junction to a high retropubic position. This action strengthens the circular fibers of the urethra.
- Many sources recommend using permanant sutures to keep the plicated fascia approximated long enough to allow secure healing.
- Leave enough fascia around and under the bladder to provide a cushion of thickness to avoid entering the bladder with suture.
- Dissect as laterally as possible to catch good specific tissue for support to the bladder neck and urethra.

---

**Author's notes**

This procedure is to correct *relaxation* of the anterior vaginal wall with or without urethrocele. Often multiple defects are present which must each be considered prior to surgery.

Removing a normal uterus to 'cure' incontinence is not necessary although many believe that one achieves better success when hysterectomy is done in conjunction with colporrhaphy procedures.

Some of the following transcriptions involve using a porcine skin collagen (Pelvicol) implant to perform an anterior and/or posterior vaginal prolapse repair. This is very useful if the cystocele or rectocele is of a severe nature. Grafts have advanced from autologous fascia and cadaveric fascia to grafts such as Repliform, DermMatrix, Pelvicol, and PelviSoft.

## ANTERIOR COLPORRHAPHY (OPERATION FOR CYSTOURETHROCELE AND KELLY URETHRAL PLICATION)

### Technique

After the patient was in the dorsolithotomy position, the patient was prepped and draped in the routine fashion. A midline incision was performed through the vaginal mucosa extending from the apex of the vagina to the urethral meatus. The flaps of the vagina were dissected laterally with sharp knife dissection. The periurethral and perivesical fascia were mobilized widely by blunt finger dissection using a single layer of gauze sponge. Entry into the white-appearing avascular plane just beneath the vaginal mucosa facilitated fascial mobilization, which was extended to the most lateral aspects of the urethral and bladder base. From a point less than 1 cm from the urethral meatus, successively vertical mattress sutures were made in the periurethral fascia. Bites were taken parallel to and on each side of the urethra to draw the fascia firmly beneath it. _____ (#2-0) sutures were used on a small curved needle. At the urethrovesical junction, the periurethral fascia was drawn carefully from its most lateral margin to add additional support to the posterior urethra.

The bladder neck suture began with a firm bite in the periurethral fascia. The suture was crossed under the urethra to anchor securely in the opposite pubourethral ligament high on the posterior aspect of the symphysis pubis. A similar suture was placed in opposite periurethral fascia and pubourethral ligament, which provided additional support to the posterior urethra and reinforced the high retropubic placement of the urethra. When the plication sutures were being placed along the course of the urethra and bladder neck, the assistant inverted the posterior floor of the urethra slightly with a Kelly clamp as each suture was tied. Cystocele was repaired by similar series of _____ (#2-0) plication sutures, which were placed in the mobilized perivesical fascia. The bladder base was displaced by a Kelly clamp and the sutures were tied in the midline.

The excess vaginal mucosa was excised and the margins of the vagina were approximated in the midline using _____ (#2-0 Ethibond) sutures. The adjacent fascia beneath the urethra and bladder was included in each bite of the vaginal suture so as to obliterate any dead space beneath the vaginal wall.

_____ inch iodoform packing was placed in the vagina. Instruments, needle, sponge, and lap counts were all correct. Estimated blood loss was _____ .

The patient tolerated the procedure well and hemostasis was judged to be excellent.

## ANTERIOR AND POSTERIOR IMPLANT COLPORRHAPHY

### Technique

The anterior vaginal skin edges were undermined until the uterosacral ligaments were located. The _____ (Pelvicol, Repliform, PelviSoft, DermMatrix, or cadaveric fascia lata) implant is anchored at five points with _____ (2-0 Ethibond). Repair of the rectoenterocele with another collagen implant was performed in similar manner by exposing the recto-enterocele and using 7 points of attachment for the posterior repair. These formed an excellent roof for the bladder and floor for the rectum. After each were tied into place, liberal irrigation was performed. The result was excellent and excess vaginal mucosa was excised then reapproximated using _____ (interrupted or continuous) suture of _____ (2-0 Ethibond on a CT-2 needle). The cystoscope was inserted into the urethra and the bladder was examined and found to be free of any injury. Suprapubic catheter was placed without complication. Estimated blood loss was _____ . The patient's condition was _____ (excellent) at the completion of the surgery.

## ABDOMINAL OR LAPAROSCOPIC SACRAL COLPOPEXY: ABDOMINAL SACRAL COLPOPEXY

### Technique

The patient was prepped and draped in the usual manner in the lithotomy position with legs in place. Pelvic examination was performed and the vaginal vault demonstrated the defects of lack of vaginal support. (There appeared to be very little, if any rectocele component, and the bladder seemed to be well supported. Most of the prolapse was along the posterior aspect of the vagina with an enterocele component.)

After the patient was prepped with Betadine from the lower ribcage and the entire abdomen, anterior thighs, perineum, vagina, and perianal area, the patient was draped to allow easy access to the vagina and lower abdomen. A Foley catheter was placed after the Betadine prep. A sponge stick with two 4 × 4 sponges was placed into the vagina and covered with sterile drapes.

A _____ abdominal incision was performed and carried down through the subcutaneous tissue to the fascia. Hemostasis was brought about using electrocautery. (The fascia can be incised and, using a sterile measuring device, a 2.5 × 10 cm strip of fascia can be excised along the fascial incision and placed between sponges moistened with saline. This can be done if synthetic graft is not available: otherwise, include transcription of graft below.) The peritoneal cavity was entered using hemostats and Metzenbaum scissors. The upper abdomen was explored. The bowel and viscera were placed up into the upper abdomen and a Balfour self-retaining retractor was inserted. The sponge forceps were then manipulated through the introitus so that the vaginal cuff could be elevated and the vaginal apex could be observed very easily in the pelvis. Allis forceps were used to grasp each lateral angle of the vagina and the vesical peritoneum overlying the vaginal apex was incised. The bladder was freed from the anterior vaginal wall and the rectum was freed from the posterior vaginal wall so that at least 3–4 cm of vaginal wall could be noted in the apex exposed. The edges of the vaginal mucosa were approximated from side to side with #2-0 delayed absorbable sutures. Some of the peritoneum and its lining were excised along with excess posterior vaginal wall and further obliterated by the Moschcowitz culdoplasty using #2-0 Prolene suture. Care was taken to pick up the uterosacral ligaments with each bite. Care was also taken to avoid placing the suture too deep so that the ureter could be avoided. Four #2-0 figure-of-eight Tevdek sutures were placed in the thickness of the vaginal wall at the apex in a single row from one lateral fornix to the other. The _____ (Pelvicol or Repliform) graft was slid down the sutures to the vaginal apex and the sutures were then tied and cut. A second row of #2-0 Vicryl sutures was then placed through the graft and into the posterior vaginal wall near the apex.

The completion of the Moschcowitz culdoplasty was completed using #2-0 Tevdek, beginning at the bottom of the cul-de-sac, and exercising care to include remnants of uterosacral ligaments in the posterior vagina but only peritoneum laterally. Only shallow bites of serosa of the sigmoid colon were carried out. There were no defects during the closure of the cul-de-sac that appeared could cause any bowel entrapment. There were no constrictions on the sigmoid colon.

With the sigmoid colon retracted to the left, the posterior and parietal peritoneum overlaying the anterior sacrum was opened longitudinally in the middle from the sacral promontory caudally to a point below S-3. The posterior sacral fascia was exposed by blunt and sharp dissection, exercising care to avoid injury to the pre-sacral vessels. A straight In-Fast drill was used to place at least two titanium screws into the caudal end of the graft through to the periosteum of the sacrum approximately 1 cm apart in the midline overlying S1 and S4 vertebrae. (*If no drill is available, then transcribe the following;* 'Three permanent sutures of #2-0 Tevdek were placed in the periosteum of the sacrum about 1 cm apart in the midline overlying S1 and S4 vertebrae. #2-0 Vicryl sutures were also utilized in between these sutures. These were on MO-4 needles and could obtain deeper bites into the periosteum of the sacrum.') The fascial graft that was attached to the vaginal apex was measured and trimmed to reach the exposed anterior sacrum without tension. (*If no drill is available, then transcribe the following;* 'The sutures in the sacrum were then placed securely in the sacral end in the fascial graft and then tied.') The graft segments were sutured to underlying sigmoid serosa and culdoplasty peritoneum to avoid any bridging between the graft and underlying tissues. This was performed with 2-0 chromic suture. The area was irrigated very thoroughly and the retroperitoneal space was reapproximated with 2-0 delayed absorbable suture.

The peritoneum was closed with #2-0 delayed absorbable suture. (The space of Retzius was not entered because an anterior repair had already previously been performed and the patient had not complained of any urinary symptoms.) A #2-0 Prolene suture was placed in a continuous suture in the fascia to approximate closing the incision. The subcutaneous tissue was closed with 3-0 plain suture after irrigation and after placing two interrupted sutures of 2-0 Vicryl in each side of the fascia following the Prolene closure. Skin was reapproximated with 5-0 Vicryl in a continuous subcuticular fashion and the incision was wiped clean with a wet lap/dry lap and benzoin applied. Steri-strips were applied and then bandage was applied.

Following placement of the bandage over the abdominal skin closure, the vaginal area was examined again. (It was noted that there would be no need for posterior colporrhaphy in that there was very little, if any, rectocele component.) The correction of vaginal prolapse and correct angle was noted to be excellent following the colpopexy. The 4 × 4 sponges were removed before and after inspection of the vagina. The patient was then removed to the Recovery Room in good condition. Estimated blood loss was approximately _____ . The patient went to the Recovery Room in good condition.

---

**Author's notes**

In-Fast straight drill can be obtained from American Medical Systems, Minnetonka, MN). Keep in mind the complications that can quickly turn this procedure into a disaster:

(1) Hemorrhage along the middle sacral artery and vessels of the sacrum – keep bone wax and sterile thumb tacks on the back table in case these are needed to control bleeding.
(2) Vaginal mesh erosion occurs within 5–9 years in 3.3% of patients.
(3) Enterocele can be prevented by use of the Moschowitz or Halbane procedure.

## ABDOMINAL REPAIR OF ENTEROCELE (MOSCHOWITZ OPERATION OR HALBANE PROCEDURE)

### Technique

With the patient in Trendelenburg position, the intestines were held back with damp packs for optimal exposure.

A purse-string suture using #0 _____ (silk or 2-0 Ethibond) suture was placed around the base of the sac to encircle the cul-de-sac of Douglas. The peritoneum was picked up in each bite, taking only light superficial bites into the serosa of the rectum. Successive purse-string sutures were placed until the uterosacral ligaments were reached; then, very firm bites were placed along these ligaments and the posterior surface of the vagina. The last suture was placed without undue tension.

The anatomical defect was completely obliterated without inclusion or injury to ureters.

### Author's notes

If the uterus is retained, it is held up and forward with a traction suture. If the uterus is absent, the posterior wall of the vaginal vault is held under traction with Allis clamps.

If a Halbane procedure is performed, the same protocol is transcribed, except that the suture placement at the base of the cul-de-sac is parallel rather than circular to close the pouch of Douglas.

## VAGINAL REPAIR OF ENTEROCELE

### Technique

After prep and drape, a midline incision was performed posteriorly, as in a posterior colporrhaphy. A tunnel was made beneath the vaginal mucosa using Metzenbaum scissors then the vagina was incised in the midline. The vagina was dissected laterally until rectocele component was exposed on both sides and the enterocele presented itself as a peritoneal pouch.

The enterocele sac was dissected free using blunt and sharp dissection. A purse-string suture using #0 _____ (silk or 2-0 Ethibond ) suture was placed on the outside of the sac at the neck. The purse-string suture was placed along the inside of the sac above the levator hiatus. An additional purse-string suture above the initial suture was also placed, incorporating bites into the uterosacral ligaments and providing additional support to the hernial repair. After all the purse-strings were tied, the margins of the sac were trimmed.

The posterior margin of the vagina was then pulled forward to place maximum tension on the uterosacral ligaments. The ligaments were approximated in the midline with two interrupted sutures that included a bite of the stump of the ligated hernial sac.

---

**Author's notes**

This procedure provides a firm new base for the cul-de-sac but if a rectocele, cystocele, or relaxed vaginal outlet is present, it should be repaired prior to completion of closure.

A small plug of Marlex mesh or synthetic graft (Pelvichol, Repliform, PelviSoft, or other) can be incorporated into the hernial defect for further strength. However, make sure prophylactic antibiotic therapy is given preoperatively and consider postoperatively.

---

## LEFORT PROCEDURE

The LeFort procedure is a very selective procedure that may be performed on elderly females without sexual activity. It involves partial colpocleisis and provides a procedure that is not too complicated and is usually done on a patient that will more than likely not tolerate too much anesthesia or complicated surgery. It is essentially an A&P (anterior and posterior) colporrhaphy with the vaginal walls sutured together closing the vagina but does not include the anterior one-third of the vagina.

---

**Technique**

With the patient in the dorsal lithotomy position, careful examination under anesthesia was completed. (*At this point, the labia can be anchored laterally with interrupted 2-0 synthetic absorbable sutures if redundant.*) The cervix was grasped with a Jacobs (or thyroid) clamp tenaculum and prolapsed from the vagina. Using a permanent marking pen, the area was outlined along the anterior and posterior vaginal mucosa that was to be undermined and removed. A scalpel was used to incise the posterior vaginal mucosa transversely at its junction with the cervix. Curved Mayo scissors were inserted underneath the posterior vaginal mucosa on top of the perirectal fascia and the vaginal mucosa was freed to the lateral margins of the marked area. The posterior vaginal mucosa was then cut along the prescribed marking lines with the curved Mayo scissors and removed.

A similar incision was carried out in the anterior vaginal mucosa at its junction with the cervix. The blades of the curved Mayo scissors were inserted underneath the anterior vaginal mucosa to dissect laterally and upward toward the urethral meatus until the limits of the marked area are reached. This procedure was facilitated by holding traction with the _____ (Jacobs, thyroid) tenaculum. The anterior vaginal mucosa was removed from the underlying pubovesical cervical fascia.

Anteriorly, the pubovesical cervical fascia was approximated to the perirectal fascia posteriorly with Lembert inverting sutures. As the suture was tied, a tunnel was created along each lateral margin for drainage of the cervical mucus to prevent the formation of a mucocele. Several sutures were placed to complete the tunnel.

Lembert _____ (0 absorbable) sutures were placed from the pubovesical cervical fascia anteriorly to the perirectal fascia posteriorly over the portio of the cervix. After several of these sutures were placed, the portio of the cervix was inverted. After several rows of sutures were completed, the cervix was totally inverted and the pubovesical and perirectal cervical fascia were plicated anteriorly and posteriorly.

A final row of _____ (0 synthetic absorbable) sutures were placed between the remaining vaginal mucosa anteriorly and posteriorly. A small wire probe could be inserted into the tunnel laterally on each side.

The vaginal mucosal sutures were completed, purposely omitting the urethra, urethrovesical angle, and posterior fourchette. (*The finished operation should result in a slight urethrocele or bulge but no attempt to close off the entire vagina should be made as this may lead to postoperative urinary incontinence.*)

## MANCHESTER-FOTHERGILL PROCEDURE

The Manchester-Fothergill procedure can be performed if there is good uterine support but prolapse of the cervix, anterior vagina, and posterior vagina. The procedure is essentially an A&P colporrhaphy with amputation of the cervix. The main advantage is that the surgeon does not have to enter the peritoneum, Operating Room time is reduced, and there is an associated low morbidity. It is ideal for the elderly patient with no other uterine disease.

### Technique

Examination under anesthesia was performed with the patient in the dorsolithotomy position. The anterior lip of the cervix was grasped with _____ (a Jacobs, thyroid) clamp and downward traction on the cervix exposed the junction of the vagina and cervix where a 360° circumferential incision was made. The bladder was sharply and bluntly dissected from the lower uterine segment up to the vesicouterine fold that was picked up and opened. The anterior cul-de-sac was opened and a finger was inserted so that the fundus and adnexa could be explored.

A right-angle Heaney retractor was placed in the anterior cul-de-sac, allowing elevation of the bladder and ureter. The cervix was rotated anteriorly, and the posterior cul-de-sac was exposed. The peritoneum of the posterior cul-de-sac was picked up and opened so that a finger could be inserted and the area explored. The uterosacral and cardinal ligaments were exposed and a _____ (Z-clamp or Heaney clamp) was placed along these ligaments bilaterally, cut, and sutured with _____ (#1 synthetic absorbable) suture.

The cervix was amputated in a wedge shape at the lower edge of the lower uterine segment with a _____ (scalpel or Bovie). The lower uterine segment was moved posteriorly; cardinal and uterosacral ligaments were brought across the anterior surface of the cervix and sutured to the lower uterine segment with interrupted _____ (#1 synthetic absorbable) sutures. The bladder and ureters were elevated out of the surgical field with the right-angle Heaney retractor. The left cardinal and uterosacral ligaments were sutured in place, overlapping those from the right side and creating a firm ligament band in front of the lower uterine segment. The lower uterine segment was held posteriorly, bringing the fundus anteriorly.

Anterior repair is performed at this time (*see this transcription*) and the vaginal mucosa was closed with _____ (#1 synthetic absorbable) sutures. A row of interrupted synthetic absorbable sutures closing the vaginal mucosa was extended to the opposite side.

A Foley catheter is placed overnight and possibly longer if a Kelly plication and/or anterior repair is performed in conjunction with the Manchester operation. If these were not performed, a catheter is not necessary.

## SACRAL SPINOUS LIGAMENT SUSPENSION

See pages 155–160.

## POSTERIOR INTRAVAGINAL SLING

See pages 151–152.

## POSTERIOR COLPORRHAPHY

See pages 149–150.

# Posterior colporrhaphy (repair of rectocele and perineal repair)

## Technique

Following proper prep and drape, the perineal skin was excised horizontally along the vaginal outlet. A midline vertical incision was initiated in the center of the mucosal edge by tunneling beneath the posterior mucosa with Metzenbaum scissors, incising the free mucosa in the midline and extending the dissection to the apex of the vagina. In a manner similar to an anterior repair, traction was placed on the upper margin of each segment of the mucosal dissection using Allis clamps. The lower margins of the incision were held under tension with additional clamps while the mucosa was separated with Metzenbaum scissors from the underlying fascia. When the midline incision was completed, the vaginal mucosa was separated laterally from the perirectal fascia and muscle attachments by sharp dissection, taking care to avoid penetrating the thin mucosa. The lateral dissection was extended as far as possible to mobilize the perirectal fascia and to expose the medial margins of the levator ani muscles. The terminal ends of the bulbocavernosus and transverse perinei muscles were also freed from the mucosa in the lower vagina.

The perirectal fascia was then drawn over the bulging rectocele using as many vertical mattress sutures of _____ (2-0 Ethibond) suture as were necessary to reinforce and completely close the hernial space over the rectal wall. The defect was sutured with certainty during this movement. Interrupted sutures of _____ (2-0 Ethibond) suture were placed deeply in the margins of the levator muscles, approximating the muscles and fascia sufficiently over the lower rectal wall to produce the desired support to the perineal body and posterior vaginal wall.

After extra-vaginal mucosa had been excised, the margins were closed, beginning in the apex of the vagina. This was done with continuous lock stitch of _____ (2-0 delayed absorbable) suture, incorporating the underlying fascia with running suture to obliterate the dead space between the vaginal wall and rectum. When the continuous mucosal suture reached the levator muscles, the deep interrupted sutures were tied. After a few supporting plication sutures were placed in the fascia and underlying muscles of the perineal body, the mucosal suture was continued over the perineum as subcuticular stitch using _____(4-0 or 5-0 delayed

153

absorbable) suture on a small curved cutting needle. The perineal muscle sutures, including the lower margins of the bulbocavernosus and the transverse perineum muscles, gave good support to the levator hiatus and pelvic floor. The result was good. Hemostasis was judged to be excellent and the patient left the Operating Room in stable condition. Instrument, needle, lap and sponge counts were all correct.

# Posterior intravaginal slingplasty

## Overview

This technique was developed to replace the sacral colpopexy and/or sacrospinous ligament suspension. Both of these invasive conventional procedures have specific risks. The sacral colpopexy procedure runs the risks of injury to the middle sacral arteries/stress urinary incontinence/mesh erosion and/or ureteral damage. Sacrospinous suspension, specifically, can cause pudendal artery and/or pudendal nerve injury, along with possible deviation of vaginal apical anatomy. On the other hand, 15–20 minute outpatient posterior intravaginal slingplasty (PIVS) can be performed under local or regional anesthesia, with the rare complication of injury to the rectum.

PIVS is indicated for apical prolapse. Disruption of the cardinal–uterosacral complex may result in uterine descensus or vaginal vault (apical) prolapse. Pregnancy, childbirth, and even the aging process can initiate weakening and stretching or tearing of the pelvic ligaments and related connective tissues, ultimately leading to uterine and/or vaginal vault prolapse. Failure to reattach the cardinal–uterosacral ligaments to the reapproximated vaginal cuff (pubocervical fascia anteriorly and rectovaginal fascia posteriorly) is a common cause of vaginal vault prolapse. An enterocele (true pelvic hernia) may form if the cuff closure does not incorporate the epithelium, pubocervical, and rectovaginal fascia.

---

### Pearls

- Cure rates are 90%.
- EBL is usually 75 ml or less.
- Most cases (90%) of PIVS vault repair are combined with graft-augmented rectocele repair in that the PIVS mesh tape is attached to the top of the graft (porcine dermal or polypropylene mesh), which is fixed to the top of the vagina.
- It is suggested that the patient undergo bowel prep with Fleet Phospho-soda and three doses of neomycin (500 mg) despite the low risk of bowel perforation.

---

## Technique

The patient was prepped and draped in the usual manner, with special attention to the vagina and buttocks. A 3–4 cm vertical incision was made in the vaginal epithelium of the posterior wall and the epithelium was dissected off the underlying rectovaginal fascia. The dissection was taken laterally to the levators and then tunneled under the vaginal epithelium up to the apex of the vagina so that the tape would not be exposed to the vaginal incision when placed. The rectovaginal fascia and rectocele were repaired and augmented with graft per routine (*may dictate this per posterior repair with or without graft). (If enterocele is present, repair is also done at this point and dictated.*)

A 5 mm stab incision was made on each buttock approximately 2–3 cm lateral and 2–3 cm inferior to the anal verge. After placing a finger into the vagina and palpating the ischial spine and pelvic sidewall just distal to the spine (levator or iliococcygeal muscle), the tunneler *(Tyco US Surgical)* was advanced through the stab incision, into the ischiorectal fossa and up towards the apex of the vagina lateral to the levator ani muscles. The finger in the vaginal incision was palpating the tunneler on the other side of the levators to help guide it towards the ischial spine. The tunneller was then brought into the vagina with finger guidance through the iliococcygeal fascia, approximately 1 cm distal to the ischial spine. The blue, blunt-tipped stylet was reversed in the tunneler. The 8 mm mesh tape was threaded through the stylet's eyelet and pulled out with the tunneler; excess tape was left at the vaginal apex.

The procedure was repeated on the other side. Taking care to keep the tape flat, it was sutured to the apex and/or graft across the entire width of the vagina. (This provided increased surface area for attachment and avoided relying on 1 or 2 sutures placed through thin vaginal skin to provide suspension.) Before closing the vaginal incision with _____ (delayed absorbable sutures), the rectum was examined to ensure that it had not been injured and that there was no undue tension of the tape across the rectum. Excess tape at the buttock incisions was cut at the skin surface, and the incisions were closed with _____ (4-0 nylon or 3M Steri-Strips).

# Presacral neurectomy

**Author's notes**

After exploratory laparotomy has been described and transcribed, the following transcription should proceed.

**Technique**

The viscera were packed with wet lap packs and a _____ retractor was used to expose the sacral promontory. The retroperitoneal space was dissected using a vertical incision. Adventitia and adipose tissue along the retroperitoneal fat area was dissected using hemoclips and Metzenbaum scissors. Care was taken to expose both bilateral ureters, which passed over the aortic bifurcation on both sides, and these were moved out of the operative field, being careful not to denude any blood supply or tissue from around the edges of the ureters. Bleeding was brought to hemostasis with hemoclips as the adventitia was dissected away from the presacral nerve plexus. The nerve plexus was elevated with right-angle forceps and tied with a free tie along the superior edge and along the superior inferior edge with another pair of right-angle forceps. Free tie was brought around the posterior inferior edge of the presacral nerve plexus and this was also tied with _____ (0-delayed absorbable) suture.

After being tied at the superior and inferior borders, the presacral nerve plexus was excised and removed from the retroperitoneal space. Hemostasis was judged to be adequate and the retroperitoneal space and adventitia was closed with _____ (2-0 chromic or delayed absorbable) in a continuous suture. _____ (Interceed) was placed over this portion of the surgery. After packs had been removed and viscera replaced back into the anatomical position, _____ Interceed was placed under the peritoneal closure using _____ (2-0 delayed absorbable) suture, thereby decreasing the chance of any postoperative adhesions. The fascia was closed in a continuous suture of #0 _____ (delayed absorbable) suture. The skin was closed with _____ (skin staples). A bandage was applied. The patient tolerated the procedure very well.

# Sacrospinous ligament fixation

Posterior intravaginal sling is a less invasive procedure than sacral colpopexy and sacrospinous ligament fixation (SSLF) but SSLF is transcribed here for those surgeons not trained in performing the posterior sling procedure.

**Specific needs**

Miya Hook or Capio suture-capturing device (Boston Scientific/Microinvasive, Natick, MA).

**Technique**

After routine prep and drape, ligament fixation was started as the posterior vaginal wall was exposed and incised to its full thickness up to the apex through the endopelvic fascia until the rectovaginal space was entered. This was performed with Metzenbaum scissors and single-layer sponges, and was done both sharply and bluntly.

The peritoneum was then resected with the posterior vaginal mucosa. The patient's right rectovaginal space was then dissected bluntly to the level of the ischial spines, and the right descending rectal pillar was perforated bluntly and sharply so that the ischial spines and sacrospinous/coccygeal complex could be adequately visualized. The perirectal space was entered. Additional blunt sharp dissection was performed until the ischial spine and sacrospinous ligament/coccygeus muscle complex were palpated and visually identified. Under direct visualization and using a _____ (Capio suture-capturing device or Miya Hook ligature carrier) to the sacrospinous ligaments, two #2 _____ (Prolene) sutures were placed through the sacrospinous/coccygeus ligament complex, approximately 2–3 cm medial to the ischial spine. After the sutures were placed in the sacrospinous/coccygeus muscle complex and through the ligament, the correctness of their placement was tested by pulling on them firmly. These sutures were then tagged.

The sacrospinous fixation was completed utilizing a pulley and a safety stitch. The pulley stitch was placed by throwing a half-knot through the suture that was taken in the posterior vaginal apex. When the end of the suture attached to the pulley stitch was held with moderate tension, the other end of the suture was drawn out, allowing the apex to be

159

drawn snugly against the sacrospinous/coccygeal complex. The safety stitch was then tied in normal fashion. The vagina was checked and found to be slightly deviated to the right. A few _____ (2-0 chromic) sutures were placed over the area of ligament fixation and interlocked in a continuous fashion to completely close the vagina. The vagina was noted to be seen in the normal anatomical position with slight deviation to the right, and the vagina was thoroughly irrigated with a _____ (normal saline/cefamandole solution) and packed with _____ (iodoform) packing. The transurethral catheter was left to gravity. The patient tolerated the procedure well and went to the Recovery Room in good condition.

**Author's notes**

(1) Usually this procedure requires additional combination procedures such as the following transcription, see Pelvic Prolapse Procedures (A&P with Enterocele Repair).
(2) The Shutt Suture Punch System, an orthopedic instrument, has been shown to allow safe and rapid placement and retrieval of suture into the sacrospinous ligament for suspension of the vagina. The technique is described by TR Sharp in *Obstet Gynecol* 1993; **82**: 893–5.

# Sacrospinous ligament fixation with anterior and posterior colporrhaphy and with complete repair of vaginal vault

## Technique

The patient was prepped and draped in the usual manner, and a catheter was placed. A weighted speculum was placed into the vagina, and the vaginal vault prolapse was spontaneously noted to be protruding out of the introitus. Bulging cystocele, rectocele, and enterocele could be noted. The anterior colporrhaphy was performed first with the entire length of the anterior vaginal wall dissected after Neo-Synephrine injection. This was performed with Metzenbaum scissors and Allis clamps in the routine manner, pushing the cystocele away from the vaginal mucosa with a single layer of gauze sponge.

After the cystocele had been fully dissected away from the vaginal mucosa, the retropubic urethral ligaments were plicated in a manner which resituated the posterior urethral vesicle angle retropubically by pulling _____ (#1 Ethibond) sutures underneath the urethra. The remaining endopelvic fascia was then plicated in the midline, reducing the cystocele using interrupted locking sutures on _____ (2-0 Ethibond). The vaginal mucosa was trimmed away and then reapproximated with _____ (2-0 delayed absorbable) suture in the usual manner.

Ligament fixation was then commenced, as the posterior vaginal wall was exposed and incised to its full thickness up to the apex through the endopelvic fascia until the rectovaginal space was entered. This was performed with Metzenbaum scissors and single-layer sponges, and carried out both sharply and bluntly. The enterocele sac was grasped with a Kelly clamp and opened into the peritoneum. The ureters were located, palpated, and avoided. The peritoneum was repaired with a highly placed purse-string suture in the routine manner.

The peritoneum was then resected with the posterior vaginal mucosa. The patient's right rectovaginal space was then dissected bluntly to the level of the ischial spines, and the right descending rectal pillar was perforated bluntly and sharply so that the ischial spines and sacrospinous/coccygeal complex could be adequately visualized. The perirectal space was entered. Additional blunt sharp dissection was performed until the ischial spine and sacrospinous ligament/coccygeus muscle complex were palpated and visually identified. Under direct visualization and using a _____ (Capio suture-capturing device or Miya Hook ligature carrier) to the sacrospinous ligaments, two _____ (#2 Prolene or Ethibond) sutures were placed through the sacrospinous/coccygeus ligament complex, approximately 2–3 cm medial to the ischial spine. After the sutures were placed in the sacrospinous/coccygeus muscle complex and through the ligament, the correctness of their placement was tested by pulling on them firmly. These sutures were then tagged.

The rectocele was then repaired by performing an excision along the peritoneal skin, and then horizontally along the vaginal outlet. Midline vertical incision was initiated in the center of the mucosal edge by tunneling beneath the posterior mucosa with Metzenbaum scissors and incising the free mucosa in the midline and extending the dissection to the apex of the vagina, incorporating the defect of the rectocele bilaterally and at the apex.

In a manner similar to the anterior repair, traction was placed on the upper margin of each segment of mucosal dissection using Allis clamps. The lower margins of the incisions were held under tension with additional clamps while the mucosa was separated with Metzenbaum scissors from the underlying fascia. When the midline incision was completed, the vaginal mucosa was separated laterally from the perineal fascia and muscle attachments by sharp dissection, taking care to avoid penetrating the mucosa. The lateral dissection was extended as far as possible to mobilize the perirectal fascia and expose the medial margins of the levator and muscles. These were already exposed from the dissection in the rectovaginal space during the _____ (Capio suture-capturing device or Miya Hook) suspension. The terminal ends of the bulbocavernosus and transverse perineal muscles were also freed from the mucosa and the lower vagina. The perirectal fascia was then drawn over the bulging rectocele, using as many vertical mattress sutures of _____ (#2-0 Ethibond) sutures as were necessary to reinforce and completely close the hernial space of the rectal wall. Interrupted sutures of _____ (#2-0 Ethibond) suture were placed deeply in the margin of the levator muscles, approximating the muscles and fascia sufficiently over the lower rectal wall to produce the desired support for the perineal body and posterior vaginal wall. After the extravaginal mucosa had been excised, the margins were closed, beginning at the apex of the vagina. This was performed with continuous lock-suture of _____ (0 delayed absorbable) suture, incorporating the underlying fascia and running suture to obliterate the dead space between the vagina and rectum. When the continuous mucosal sutures were completed and the levator muscles reached, the deep interrupted sutures were tied. After a few supporting plication sutures were placed in the fascia and underlying muscles of the perineal body, the mucosal suture was continued over the perineum as a subcuticular stitch using a _____ (4-0 or 5-0 delayed absorbable) suture on a small, curved cutting needle. The perineal muscle sutures, including the lower margins of the bulbocavernosus and transverse perinei muscles, gave good support to the levator hiatus and pelvic floor. The result was good. Hemostasis was judged to be excellent.

The sacrospinous fixation was completed utilizing a pulley and a safety stitch. The pulley stitch was placed by throwing a half-knot through the suture that was taken in the posterior vaginal apex. When the end of the suture attached to the pulley stitch was held with moderate tension, the other end of the suture was drawn out, allowing the apex to be drawn snugly against the sacrospinous/coccygeal complex. The safety stitch was then tied in normal fashion. The vagina was checked and found to be slightly deviated to the right. A few _____ (2-0 chromic) sutures were placed over the area of ligament fixation and interlocked in a continuous fashion to completely close the vagina. The vagina was noted to be seen in the normal anatomical position with slight deviation to the right, and the vagina was thoroughly irrigated with a _____ (normal saline/cefamandole solution) and packed with _____ (iodoform) packing. The transurethral catheter was left to gravity. The patient tolerated the procedure well and went to the Recovery Room in good condition.

---

**Author's note**

The Shutt Suture Punch System, an orthopedic instrument, has been shown to allow safe and rapid placement and retrieval of suture into the sacrospinous ligament for suspension of the vagina. This technique is described by TR Sharp in *Obstet Gynecol* 1993; **82**: 893–5.

# Salpingectomy

## Technique

After the patient had been placed in the supine position and routine prep and drape had been performed, the incision was made and was carried down through the subcutaneous fat to the fascia. Hemostasis was obtained, utilizing hemostats and electrocautery. The fascia was incised with the scalpel blade and extended with Mayo scissors. The midline was opened between the two rectus sheaths and the peritoneum was picked up with two hemostats and with the scalpel blade. The peritoneum was then extended with the Metzenbaum scissors and an _____ (O'Sullivan or Balfour) retractor was placed in the peritoneal cavity. Necessary exposure was obtained and _____ (describe the findings).

The above findings being noted, neither salpingotomy, manual expression, nor segmental resection could be performed. The affected fallopian tube was elevated and the mesosalpinx were clamped with a succession of Kelly clamps at the serosa of the tube, as close as possible to the tube. The tube was then excised by cutting a small myometrial wedge at the uterine cornu. Figure-of-eight sutures of 0 _____ (delayed absorbable) material were used to close the myometrium at the site of the wedge resection. The mesosalpinx was closed with interrupted sutures of 0 _____ (delayed absorbable) suture. Complete hemostasis was noted. The fundus was held forward and the round and broad ligaments were sutured over the uterine cornu in a modified Coffey technique, accomplishing complete peritonealization. Mattress sutures anchored the broad ligament to the uterus. A 0 _____ (delayed absorbable) suture was used to penetrate the broad ligament from its anterior surface just below the round ligaments, approximately 2–3 cm from the cornua. The second bite was taken into the fundus of the uterus, slightly posterior and superior to the uterine incision. The suture was then placed through the posterior aspect of the broad ligament, approximately 1 cm lateral to the previous suture. After this suture was tied, the cornual incision in the mesosalpinx was peritonealized. There was no excessive tension on this suture and supporting sutures were placed in the myometrium and the round ligament to be certain that peritonealization would remain in place. Hemostasis was judged to be excellent.

After thorough irrigation of the peritoneal cavity, Kelly clamps were used on the edges of the peritoneum so as to close the peritoneum in a continuous suture of 2-0 _____ . Three-point suturing was used to avert the cut peritoneal edges and make the intraperitoneal suture line as smooth as possible. Fascial edges were approximated following reapproximation of the rectus sheath with a single suture of #1 _____ in a continuous fashion. The subcutaneous layer was irrigated thoroughly and then approximated with continuous sutures of 3-0 _____ on a _____ needle. The skin was reapproximated in the routine fashion and the patient left the Operating Room in stable condition.

# Salpingotomy (linear)

**Technique**

(Describe the laparotomy portion and findings.) The affected fallopian tube was exposed, elevated, and stabilized. A linear incision was made with _____ (scalpel or laser) over the distended segment of the tube. The incision was extended through the antimesenteric wall until entry was made into the lumen of the distended ova duct. Gentle pressure was then exerted from the opposite side of the fallopian tube. The products of gestation were gently expressed from the lumen. Gentle traction with forceps without teeth and gentle suction were used but care was taken to avoid trauma to the mucosa. Remaining fragments of the anchoring trophoblast were removed by profuse irrigation of the lumen with warm Ringer's lactate solution. Small tubal vessels were easily identified while the fallopian tube was being irrigated and complete hemostasis to tubal mucosa was brought into effect utilizing an ophthalmological cautery.

Mucosal margins were then closed with interrupted sutures of 7-0 _____ (delayed absorbable) suture, making sure that only the serosa and muscularis were approximated without undue tension. Care was taken to ensure that no suture material was retained on the mucosal surface. After hemostasis was judged to be adequate, the abdomen was explored for extra blood clots and these were all removed. Proper irrigation was performed and the peritoneum was closed along the posterior rectus sheath with a continuous suture of 2-0 _____ suture. Three-point suture was used to avert cut peritoneal edges to make the intraperitoneal suture line as smooth as possible. The bilateral rectus sheath muscles were reapproximated with interrupted _____ sutures. The fascia was then reapproximated with single sutures of #1 _____ in a continuous fashion. The subcutaneous fat was reapproximated with 3-0 _____ . The skin was then reapproximated and a bandage was applied. The patient was removed to the Recovery Room in stable condition.

**Author's notes**

When closing the mucosal margins, it is optional to use no suture, thus leaving the tube open.

# Sterilization procedures

## Overview

As important as operative transcription, other documentation in regards to sterilization is very important. During history, operative, or discharge notes it might be useful as a guideline to document the following:

(1) The patient understands that she will be permanently unable to bear children, even though the success rate of subsequent reversal might be high.

(2) She understands that effectiveness is not guaranteed and that a failure rate of 5 per 1000 procedures is known to occur with the commonly performed procedures.

(3) Operative and anesthetic complications such as hemorrhage, bowel, ureteral, and bladder damage have been explained to the patient and she understands, including the possibility of death (1 out of 30 000 procedures).

(4) Explanation of the various methods available is understood by the patient and she has chosen _____ . (Document if she was given a pamphlet or if she was allowed to view a video demonstrating the various methods.)

(5) The patient has had it pointed out to her that technical problems or complications can turn a laparoscopy into a laparotomy (in particular, mention this in conjunction with patients that may have had prior abdominal or pelvic surgery).

(6) Be sure the consent is clear, specific, and spells out *permanent* results but that *failure is possible.*

(7) Perform the surgery early in the patient's cycle, perform a pregnancy test, and/or inform the patient about the possibility of pregnancy at the time of interval sterilization. Advise and document that the patient understands the possibility of ectopic pregnancy following tubal ligation (half the pregnancies that follow tubal ligation are ectopic) and that she needs to report any symptoms of pregnancy!

---

**Important points/pearls**

- Most failures with clips occur when the clip is placed too distal on the tube or at oblique angles to the axis of the tube. Make certain that the Hulka clip is within 3 cm of the uterus but not too close either in that at least 3 cm of isthmus next to the uterus will minimize the chance of uteroperitoneal fistula and, in turn, an ectopic pregnancy.

- A Falope ring can fail if not enough tube is drawn into the ring, so make certain there is an adequate loop of tube above the band.

- If video equipment is available for video laparoscopic documentation, use it. Of course, this medicolegal documentation can backfire in court if the technique is documented as poor and the patient is pregnant. Video would most definitely be helpful if a repeat procedure is necessary.

- Avoid using single rather than double ligatures. Avoid techniques such as the Madlener technique (not described in this book because of its high failure rate).

- If colpotomy is performed, use prophylactic antibiotics or simply avoid this method because tubal occlusion performed through the vagina has been associated with a higher rate of pelvic abscess and other complications in the past.

- Be familiar with the institutional bipolar equipment. Use waveform rather than coagulation or blended form. Use a power setting of at least 25 W. Coagulate at least 3 cm of tube and/or transect the tube to decrease the possibility of pregnancy.

- Pathology specimens are not necessary to prove occlusion and may increase the possibility of complications, but if a pathology report is ordered, make certain that it is given full attention. A hysterosalpingogram might be helpful postoperatively to document tubal occlusion if a full lumen has not been documented by the pathologist.

---

## HYSTEROSCOPIC SILICONE PLUG TECHNIQUE

See the Hysteroscopic sterilization (Essure) chapter. Below is a very similar technique using the silicone plug rather than the small metal implants, as in the Essure kit.

## Technique

Bimanual vaginal examination was performed so that the size of the uterus and orientation of the uterine corpus in relation to the cervix was determined.

After routine scrubbing, gloving, prepping, and draping – a speculum was inserted and the cervix and vagina were again disinfected over a wide area. (If paracervical anesthesia is used – describe here.) The optical assembly was mounted on the instrument with care so as not to soil the optics and sleeves. Initially, the _____ flow rate was set at _____ . (For $CO_2$ this rate is 75 ml/min but Dextran 70 is the distention medium currently being used in the Netherlands.)

A single-tooth tenaculum was used to grasp the anterior lip of the cervix and traction with the left hand corrected for proper vaginal axis.

The end of the hysteroscope was inserted so as to examine the plicae palmatae which appeared _____ (essentially normal if so). The lens then came in contact with the internal os and, after approximately 15–20 seconds, the _____ ($CO_2$) pressure dilated the orifice and the hysteroscope was then advanced to the center of the orifice. The instrument was then advanced into the uterine cavity without injury or complication.

The flow rate of _____ (30 ml/min for $CO_2$) was then adjusted for the remainder of the procedure. The uterine cavity was explored in a systematic manner, examining the anterior, posterior, sidewalls, fundus, and cornua. (Describe any significant findings or state that all was normal in that PID is a contraindication for this procedure.)

The disposable catheter from the Ovabloc kit was placed through the operative channel of the hysteroscope and the catheter was placed into the ostium of the right fallopian tube. The radiopaque silicone monomer was then injected into the right fallopian tube until complete plugging was apparent. The same procedure was performed on the left tube. Examination revealed no perforation of the uterine fundus and no apparent injury to any pelvic organs.

Instrumentation was removed from the cervix and vagina. The patient was in stable condition. The patient was advised to undergo pelvic X-ray in 3 months prior to coitus without contraception. She was alert and understood these instructions prior to discharge.

**Author's notes**

Determine that the patient is in the first half of her menstrual cycle (this is the best time to perform hysteroscopy in that the uterine mucosa is thin and the internal cervical os is easier to pass and there is no risk of pregnancy).

This procedure has not been approved by the Food and Drug Administration (FDA), except for research use as a permanent method, as of publication of this book. It is not recommended until all study results in regards to the use of the silicone catalytic polymerization in situ have been fully evaluated. Although this method is promising for the future, since it is investigational, this point should certainly be explained to the patient and all aspects documented in full detail if this technique is used at this time. Essure is approved and can be found under hysteroscopy.

## IRVING STERILIZATION

**Technique**

Following routine prep, drape, and _____ (laparotomy or mini-laparotomy), the right fallopian tube was located and doubly ligated with #2-0 _____ approximately 3 cm from the uterine cornu and then severed. The sutures on the proximal end of the tube were left long. This tubal stump was then dissected free from the mesosalpinx and mobilized. A small nick was made in the serosa on the posterior surface of the uterus near the cornu in as avascular an area as could be found and musculature was penetrated with a mosquito clamp for approximately 1 cm and with the clamp spread sufficiently to admit the tube. The fallopian tube and one of the ligatures attached to the tubal stump was threaded with a round needle. Guided by a groove director, the needle was thrust to the bottom of the pocket created by the mosquito clamp and carried out to the uterine surface. The other suture attached to the tubal stump was treated in a similar manner, bringing it to the surface of the uterus about 1 cm from the first suture. Traction was exerted on the sutures and tubal stump was buried in the uterine musculature. The sutures were then tied together and a suture of fine _____ was used to close the edges of the pocket more tightly around the buried tube.

The same procedure was performed on the left fallopian tube in that it was doubly ligated with #2-0 _____ approximately 3 cm from the uterine cornu and then severed. The sutures of the proximal end of the fallopian tube were left long and this tubal stump was then dissected free from the mesosalpinx and mobilized. A small incision was made in the serosa on the posterior surface of the uterus near the cornu in an avascular area and the musculature was penetrated with a mosquito clamp for about 1 cm. With the clamp spread sufficiently to admit the fallopian tube, one of the ligatures attached to the tube was threaded with a round needle and was guided by a groove director and the needle was thrust to the bottom of the pocket created by the mosquito clamp and carried out to the uterine surface. The other suture attached to the tubal stump was treated in similar manner, bringing it to the surface of the uterus about 1 cm from the first suture. Traction was exerted on the sutures and the tubal stump was buried in the uterine musculature. The sutures were then tied together and suture of fine _____ was used to close the edges of the pocket more tightly about the tube.

At the completion of the sterilization, hemostasis was found to be excellent and the remainder of the operation was performed in the routine manner. Describe closure.

### Author's notes

A modified Irving operation was performed and transcribed secondary to knowledge that according to the classical Irving's original description of the operation, the ligated end of the distal portion of the fallopian tube was buried beneath the leaves of the broad ligament. The burying of this end of the tube is presently considered to be optional, because it gives a neat appearance and adds nothing to the effectiveness of the sterilization. Furthermore, it adds a slightly more dangerous step to the procedure in that a blood vessel may be nicked occasionally during this step.

### KROENER METHOD

### Author's note

The type of incision must be described in that a mini-laparotomy, laparotomy, or even colpotomy may be performed during this method of sterilization.

### Technique

Following exposure of the fimbriated end of the oviduct into the operative field, the fallopian tube was grasped with a Babcock clamp. The mesosalpinx and outer third of the fallopian tube were clamped, doubly ligated with #2 absorbable sutures twice, and excised to remove the entire fimbriated end of the fallopian tube. The outer third of the fallopian tube was grasped with a Heaney clamp, and the initial ligature was a free tie to secure the blood vessels in the mesosalpinx. A transfixing ligature through the wall of the fallopian tube was placed between the Heaney clamp and the initial ligature to completely secure the collateral circulation and to occlude the lumen of the oviduct. The fimbriated end of the tube was then excised with Metzenbaum scissors between the clamp and the outer ligature. Following the excision of the fimbria and small segment of the ampullary portion of the fallopian tube, it was noted that the entire functional component of the oviduct was completely removed.

The same procedure was performed on both fallopian tubes. Hemostasis was judged to be excellent. The incision was reapproximated in the routine fashion. All instrument counts, lap counts, and sponge counts were correct. Estimated blood loss was _____ . The patient tolerated the procedure well and went to the Recovery Room in good condition.

## LAPAROSCOPIC STERILIZATION TECHNIQUES – BILATERAL PARTIAL SALPINGECTOMY

### Technique

The patient was prepped with solution and draped in the lithotomy position with special attention to the area of the umbilicus and cervix. Weighted speculum was placed into the vagina so as to expose the cervix. A _____ tenaculum was placed into the cervix to enable the uterus to be manipulated. The weighted speculum was removed and the bladder was emptied with a catheter. Gloves were then changed prior to abdominal incision.

A small subumbilical incision was performed and _____ Verres needle was placed into the incision and checked by the syringe, the hanging drop, the bubble, and the gas pressure register methods. All methods indicated proper placement of the needle.

Pneumoperitoneum of approximately 3 liters of $CO_2$ was established; then _____ trocar was properly inserted into the abdomen. The sound of escaping gas confirmed proper location in the abdomen as the trocar was removed from the sleeve.

Fiberoptics (and video camera if available) were connected to the laparoscope and this was inserted through the sleeve under _____ (direct or video) laparoscopic visualization. Trendelenburg position was increased and approximately 1–1.5 liters more of $CO_2$ gas was allowed into the abdomen to displace the viscera, so as to easily visualize the pelvic organs. (Describe the findings.)

Laparoscopic flat duckbill bipolar forceps were brought into contact with the right fallopian tube and mesosalpinx. Coagulation and avulsion of the tube was performed for approximately 10 seconds over a distal, midportion, and proximal area of the middle one-third of the fallopian tube. The cauterized segment of the tube and mesosalpinx were then transected twice with a pair of laparoscopic hook scissors. The middle portion of this cauterized segment was removed. Hemostasis was judged to be excellent during the entire procedure. The exact same procedure was performed on the opposite left fallopian tube. Both fallopian tubes were observed to be adequately cauterized and transected. The procedure was discontinued and the abdomen was inspected. Hemostasis was excellent. There was no apparent injury to any bladder, bowel, vessels, or other visceral structures. The $CO_2$ was released from the abdominal cavity. All instrumentation was removed from the abdomen. The subumbilical incision was reapproximated with a figure-of-eight suture utilizing 3-0 _____ suture. Neosporin and Band-Aid were applied to the incision. All instrumentation was removed from the vagina and the patient went to the Recovery Room in excellent condition.

## LAPAROSCOPIC STERILIZATION TECHNIQUES – CAUTERIZATION AND TRANSECTION OF THE FALLOPIAN TUBES

### Technique

The patient was prepped and draped in the usual manner and placed in the modified lithotomy position with the legs at 45° angle axis to the table. After assuring that the patient's buttocks extended over the edge of the operating table, the table was tilted to approximately 15° of Trendelenburg's position to help the peritoneum displace the intestines out of the pelvis. With the patient properly positioned on the table, bimanual examination and vaginal cleansing was performed. The abdominal wall was scrubbed with and painted with antiseptic solution, with special attention directed around the umbilicus. The patient's bladder was emptied by catheter and a vaginal retractor was inserted. The anterior lip of the cervix was grasped with a _____ tenaculum and inserted into the uterine cavity for uterine manipulation.

The outer surgical gloves were removed and, with underlying surgical gloves in place, attention was focused on the abdominal cavity. A 2 mm skin incision was made in the lower margin of the umbilicus. A large-bore Verres needle was placed into the incision. It was inserted through the incision and passed down to the fascia while counter traction was applied by means of surgeon and assistant pressure on the skin at 5 o'clock and 7 o'clock of the incision. A quick, short plunge of the needle through the abdominal fascia and peritoneum directed toward the center of the uterus was performed and the needle was tested to determine whether it had been properly placed. The gas pressure registered by the $CO_2$ pneumoperitoneum was noted not to be elevated and then attachment of the gas tubing was performed and approximately 3 liters of gas was allowed to form a pneumoperitoneum. With the pneumoperitoneum established, the needle was withdrawn and the umbilical incision was enlarged from 2 mm to approximately 1 cm.

A laparoscopic trocar and sleeve were inserted through the incision with a twisting motion and utilizing the lifted abdomen with the assistant's hand. The trocar was inserted as far as the rectus fascia. The trocar and sleeve were then angled to a point slightly toward the pelvis and a short, quick, stabbing motion was used to penetrate the rectus fascia and peritoneum all at once. The trocar was withdrawn from its sleeve and the trumpet valve on the sleeve was depressed slightly so as to listen for the sound of gas escaping for the pneumoperitoneum. This sound confirmed that the trocar sleeve was properly located and then this was shut to ensure that the gas would no longer escape. A fiberoptic light cable was now connected to the laparoscope and the light turned on. The laparoscope was gently inserted into the trocar sleeve while watching through the eyepiece. It was inserted at an angle to the abdomen of approximately 15–20° and then advanced into the pelvis to identify the structures there. The gas hose was then connected to the gas port on the sleeve. A small amount of gas (approximately 1–1.5 liters) was allowed to flow into the abdomen to better displace the intestines out of the pelvis. The pelvis was then thoroughly inspected for visible gynecological abnormalities. (Describe findings.)

Following the laparoscopic examination, the uterus was manipulated to bring the fallopian tube on the right into view. The forceps handle was closed and this compressed the fallopian tube and simultaneously brought the flat, duckbill portion of the tips in contact with the mesosalpinx. After the first burn and avulsion of the tube, the second burn was applied to the proximal stump. The electric current was applied for approximately 10 seconds. The cauterized segment of the tube and mesosalpinx were then transected with a pair of hook scissors. Hemostasis was judged to be excellent. The same procedure was performed on the opposite fallopian tube. After both fallopian tubes were observed to be very adequately transected, the procedure was discontinued and the $CO_2$ gas was released from the abdominal cavity.

All instrumentation was removed from the abdomen. After reapproximation of the incision with 3-0 _____ , a Band-Aid was applied to the area and the instruments were removed from the vagina. The patient was removed to the Recovery Room in excellent condition.

## LAPAROSCOPIC STERILIZATION TECHNIQUES – SPRING-LOADED CLIP OR HULKA TECHNIQUE

### Technique

The patient was prepped and draped in the usual manner and placed in the modified lithotomy position with the legs at 45° angle axis to the table. After assuring that the patient's buttocks extended over the edge of the operating table, the table was tilted to approximately 15° of Trendelenburg's position to help the peritoneum displace the intestines out of the pelvis. With the patient properly positioned on the table, bimanual examination and vaginal cleansing was performed. The abdominal wall was scrubbed with _____ and painted with antiseptic solution, with special attention directed around the umbilicus. The patient's bladder was emptied by catheter and a vaginal retractor was inserted. The anterior lip of the cervix was grasped with a _____ tenaculum and inserted into the uterine cavity for uterine manipulation.

The outer surgical gloves were removed and, with underlying surgical gloves in place, attention was focused on the abdominal cavity. A 2 mm skin incision was made in the lower margin of the umbilicus. A large-bore _____ Verres needle was placed into the incision. It was inserted through the incision and passed down to the fascia while counter traction was applied by means of surgeon and assistant pressure on the skin at 5 o'clock and 7 o'clock of the incision. A quick, short plunge of the needle through the abdominal fascia and peritoneum directed toward the center of the uterus was performed and the needle was tested to determine whether it had been properly placed. The _____ test was utilized to determine proper placement. (Describe results of test.) The gas pressure registered by the $CO_2$ pneumoperitoneum was noted not to be elevated and then attachment of the gas tubing was performed and approximately 3 liters of gas was allowed to form a pneumoperitoneum. With the pneumoperitoneum established, the needle was withdrawn and the umbilical incision was enlarged from 2 mm to approximately 1 cm.

A laparoscopic _____ trocar and sleeve were inserted through the incision with a twisting motion and utilizing the lifted abdomen with the assistant's hand. The trocar was inserted as far as the rectus fascia. The trocar and sleeve were then angled to a point slightly toward the pelvis and a short, quick, stabbing motion was used to penetrate the rectus fascia and peritoneum all at once. The trocar was withdrawn from its sleeve and the trumpet valve on the sleeve was depressed slightly so as to listen for the sound of gas escaping for the pneumoperitoneum. This sound confirmed that the trocar sleeve was properly located and then this was shut to ensure that the gas would no longer escape. A fiber-optic light cable was now connected to the laparoscope and the light turned on. (Describe if the video camera is attached.) The laparoscope was gently inserted into the trocar sleeve while watching through the eyepiece (or while watching the video screen if video laparoscopy is used). The laparoscope was inserted at an angle to the abdomen of approximately 15–20° and then advanced into the pelvis to identify the structures there. The gas hose was then connected to the gas port on the sleeve. A small amount of gas (approximately 1–1.5 liters) was allowed to flow into the abdomen to better displace the intestines out of the pelvis. The pelvis was then thoroughly inspected for visible gynecological abnormalities. (Describe any abnormalities.)

Following the placement of laparoscopic instruments, the spring-loaded clip – consisting of two small serrated Silastic jaws held together by the metal clip with the teeth at the end of the jaws which locked the clip into place – was attached to the fallopian tube with an applicator. This was performed on the right fallopian tube: the same application was performed on the left tube. Following completion of the application, the instrumentation was removed from the abdomen and gas was released from the abdomen. The incision was reapproximated with 3-0 chromic in the routine manner and the instruments were also removed from the vagina. The patient went to the Recovery Room in good condition. Blood loss was minimal and counts were correct.

**Author's notes**

(1) Although the failure rate with this method (clip or Hulka) is 2%, and seems somewhat higher than with other laparoscopic sterilization methods, the damage to the tube is felt to be less and for this reason this procedure was used on this patient since she may wish to have reversal of sterilization in the future (it might be preferable to add this type of comment either in the history or operative transcription).

(2) With all laparoscopic techniques performed under *local anesthesia*, it is necessary to transcribe the type of anesthetic injected and the method used prior to the umbilical skin incision.

## LAPAROSCOPIC STERILIZATION TECHNIQUES – FALOPE RING (YOON OR SILASTIC BAND TECHNIQUE)

**Technique**

The patient was prepped and draped in the usual manner and placed in the modified lithotomy position with the legs at 45° angle axis to the table. After assuring that the patient's buttocks extended over the edge of the operating table, the table was tilted to approximately 15° of

Trendelenburg's position to help the peritoneum displace the intestines out of the pelvis. With the patient properly positioned on the table, bimanual examination and vaginal cleansing was performed. The abdominal wall was scrubbed with _____ and painted with antiseptic solution, with special attention directed around the umbilicus. The patient's bladder was emptied by catheter and a vaginal retractor was inserted. The anterior lip of the cervix was grasped with a _____ tenaculum and inserted into the uterine cavity for manipulation.

The outer surgical gloves were removed and, with underlying surgical gloves in place, attention was focused on the abdominal cavity. A 2 mm skin incision was made in the lower margin of the umbilicus. A large-bore _____ needle was placed into the incision. It was inserted through the incision and passed down to the fascia while counter traction was applied by means of surgeon and assistant pressure on the skin at 5 o'clock and 7 o'clock of the incision. A quick, short plunge of the needle through the abdominal fascia and peritoneum directed toward the center of the uterus was performed and the needle was tested to determine whether it had been properly placed. The test was utilized to determine proper placement. (Describe the results of the test.)

The gas pressure registered by the $CO_2$ pneumoperitoneum was noted not to be elevated and then attachment of the gas tubing was performed and approximately 3 liters of gas was allowed to form a pneumoperitoneum. With the pneumoperitoneum established, the needle was withdrawn and the umbilical incision was enlarged from 2 mm to approximately 1 cm.

A laparoscopic trocar and sleeve were inserted through the incision with a twisting motion and utilizing the lifted abdomen with the assistant's hand. The trocar was inserted as far as the rectus fascia. The trocar and sleeve were then angled to a point slightly toward the pelvis and a short, quick, stabbing motion was used to penetrate the rectus fascia and peritoneum all at once. The trocar was withdrawn from its sleeve and the trumpet valve on the sleeve was depressed slightly so as to listen for the sound of gas escaping for the pneumoperitoneum. This sound confirmed that the trocar sleeve was properly located and then this was shut to ensure that the gas would no longer escape. A fiberoptic light cable was now connected to the laparoscope and the light turned on. The laparoscope was gently inserted into the trocar sleeve while watching through the eyepiece. It was inserted at an angle to the abdomen of approximately 15–20° and then advanced into the pelvis to identify the structures there. The gas hose was then connected to the gas port on the sleeve. A small amount of gas (approximately 1–1.5 liters) was allowed to flow into the abdomen to better displace the intestines out of the pelvis. The pelvis was then thoroughly inspected for visible gynecological abnormalities. (Describe findings.)

Following the completion of the placement of the laparoscopic instruments, the specially equipped laparoscope, which was loaded with Silastic band (Falope ring), was inserted in standard fashion. *(Some of the newer models can accommodate two rings simultaneously, which enables the operator to apply both rings to each tube without having to bring the scope back out through the sleeve to reload. Some of the newer versions also have canals that allow optional application of local anesthetic, which may temporarily decrease postoperative discomfort. If this anesthetic is applied to the tube, it should be transcribed here.)* The tongs at the band applicator were then extended and the right fallopian tube was grasped at the ampullo-isthmic junction and brought into the applicator. The band was pushed over a knuckle of the tube and then the tongs were released and the tube was dropped into the cul-de-sac. The left fallopian tube was treated in the same manner as the right. Instrumentation was removed from the abdomen. As much $CO_2$ was removed at this time as possible. Closure of the incision was performed with 3-0 _____ . Vaginal instrumentation was removed and the patient tolerated the procedure well.

**Author's notes**

If the local anesthesia is applied to aid relief of postoperative pain after tubal sterilization with Falope rings, then insert 'each fallopian tube was sprayed with 5 ml of 0.5% bupivacaine'.

**Footnote**

The mesosalpinx of each tube can also be injected with 3–5 ml of 0.5% bupivacaine after application of the rings, but this method can increase the possibility of bleeding and has not been demonstrated to significantly reduce pain or shorten Recovery Room stays over the 'spray' method.

**Reference**

Borgatta L. *Am J Gyn Health* 1991; **5(1)**: 1.

## MINI-LAP POMEROY STERILIZATION

### Technique

Following the placement of the patient in the supine position and after proper prep and drape, a small mini-lap incision was made transversely over the suprapubic area and carried down to the subcutaneous fascia. Fascia was entered with a scalpel blade and extended with Mayo scissors and the peritoneum was grasped with two hemostats and entered with Metzenbaum scissors. The peritoneum was extended with Metzenbaum scissors and the uterus was located with the surgeon's fingers.

Following the location of the uterus, the fallopian tube was grasped with a Babcock clamp and delivered. After identification of the fimbria of the right fallopian tube, a midportion of the right fallopian tube was held up and ligated twice with a #2 plain suture. The loop was then cut off with Metzenbaum scissors and hemostasis was achieved by using electrocautery. The fallopian tube was placed back into the peritoneum and the left fallopian tube was located with the surgeon's finger and delivered through the incision with the Babcock clamp around the midportion of the fallopian tube. After identification of the fimbriated end, the loop was held up and ligated twice with an absorbable #2 plain suture. The loop was then cut off with the Metzenbaum scissors and hemostasis was achieved. The bisected tube was then placed back into the peritoneum and both portions of fallopian tube were handed off to the surgical scrub nurse.

Peritoneum was then reapproximated with a continuous absorbable suture and the fascia was reapproximated with _____ (# 2-0 Vicryl) continuous suture. The subcutaneous tissue was closed with _____ #5(0 Vicryl) suture.

A subcuticular suture was used in a continuous fashion with #5-0 _____ . The patient tolerated the procedure well and the incisional area was treated with a bandage. The patient went to the Recovery Room in good condition. Counts were correct and blood loss minimal.

### Important points/pearls

It is important to use plain suture on the tubes. Plain suture dissolves within a few days causing the ends of the tube to retract and decrease the risk of spontaneous reanastomosis.

## POSTPARTUM POMEROY STERILIZATION

### Technique

Following delivery, the patient was prepared for surgery in the routine manner. A small subumbilical incision was performed and the peritoneum easily entered. The fundus of the uterus was easily located with the surgeon's fingers through the incision and the fallopian tube was swept into view so that the midportion of the tube could be grasped with Babcock clamps and delivered. As the loop was held up, the fallopian tube was traced down to the fimbriated end to ensure that this was the fallopian tube. This was performed on the right side. The midportion of the fallopian tube was grasped again with Babcock clamps and it was ligated twice with two _____ (#2 plain absorbable) sutures. The loop was cut away with Metzenbaum scissors and hemostasis was performed using electrocautery. After completion of the operation on the right fallopian tube, the two severed ends of tube were placed back into the peritoneum so as to have a tendency to retract from one another.

The process was repeated on the opposite side, grasping the midportion of the left fallopian tube and following it to the fimbriated end to guarantee that this was the fallopian tube. The midportion was again grasped and the loop being held up was ligated with two _____ (#2 plain absorbable) sutures. The loop was cut away with Metzenbaum scissors and the fallopian tube placed back into the peritoneum following excellent hemostasis. The peritoneum and fascia were reapproximated in the usual continuous fashion, utilizing _____(#2-0 Vicryl), and the skin was reapproximated with subcuticular stitch using _____(#5-0 Vicryl). The patient's incision was cleaned and Band-Aid was placed over the incision. The patient tolerated the procedure well and was sent to the Recovery Room in good condition.

## UCHIDA MINI-LAP STERILIZATION

### Technique

After the patient was placed in the supine position, and also in modified lithotomy position, the patient was prepped and draped in the usual manner for a vaginoabdominal procedure. Following placement of the uterine manipulator in the endometrial cavity, a 1 cm suprapubic incision was made and carried down to the fascia. The fascia and peritoneum were entered and the uterine fundus was maneuvered forward by the manipulator in the uterine cavity. A Babcock clamp was then used to deliver the fallopian tube through the small incision. The right fallopian tube was located first. At its midpoint, the mesosalpinx was dissected from the overlying muscular tube. This was accomplished by injecting a sufficient amount of saline–epinephrine solution at the tubo-mesosalpingeal junction to produce ballooning of the mesosalpinx. An avascular portion of the mesosalpinx was incised with Metzenbaum scissors. The muscular tube was then grasped through this incision with the clamp and delivered into a loop, and the tube was divided. Serosa from the proximal end was stripped back by blunt dissection. A 3–5 cm segment of the fallopian tube was excised, leaving only a small stump. This proximal stump was ligated with a #2 nonabsorbable suture twice and allowed to fall back between the ballooned leaves of the broad ligament. The distal stump was then ligated and the edge of the broad ligament was closed with a suture of #3-0 that terminated with a purse-string suture around the free end of the distal tube. The suture was tied so that the distal end of the fallopian tube projected into the abdominal cavity.

The same procedure that was performed on the right fallopian tube was performed on the left fallopian tube. The incision was closed in routine manner. Counts were correct and the patient tolerated the procedure well. Estimated blood loss was minimal. The patient went to the Recovery Room in good condition.

## VAGINAL BILATERAL TUBAL STERILIZATION

This procedure was popular in the 1970s and 1980s then went out of vogue due to higher infection rates. Remember to use pre-op antibiotics for this procedure. The author prefers this method of sterilization in that it leaves no scar whatsoever and the pain is less than any of the other procedures. The author also uses metronidazole twice daily for a few days postoperatively and has never had a postoperative infection in hundreds of patients undergoing this procedure.

Make sure that PLAIN CATGUT suture is utilized when ligating fallopian tubes. This suture dissolves faster than treated chromic, semi-permanent, or permanent suture. This property is advantageous in that there is a less likely chance of spontaneous reanastomosis of the tube in that the tubal stumps separate quicker from one another.

### Specific needs

(1) Medium to small Valentine retractor
(2) Wet JET pack (McNeil #40120)
(3) Ethicon Endo-loop
(4) Long Babcock clamp.

## Technique

The patient was prepped and draped in the routine manner in Candy Cane stirrups, with the patient in a mild Trendelenburg position. A short-bladed Auvard weighted retractor was placed in the vagina. The posterior aspect of the vagina was injected with Marcaine (bupivacaine) 0.5% with epinephrine while the lower lip of the cervix was held up out of the way of the needle. A small colpotomy incision was then made with the _____ (scalpel or Bovie). Peritoneal fluid was encountered and the incision was slightly enlarged using the Mayo scissors. A long-bladed Steiner-Auvard retractor was then placed into the vagina and through the colpotomy incision into the peritoneum while the short Auvard was removed.

A Valentine retractor was placed into the peritoneum along the posterior aspect of the uterine corpus and lifted to the right side of the patient. The left fallopian tube and left ovary fell easily into view. The fimbria could be identified, which insured that the structure that appeared to be fallopian tube was fallopian tube. The fallopian tube was grasped in the middle third with a Babcock clamp and an Endo-loop with _____ (0 to 2-0 plain) suture was placed around the Babcock clamp and the suture was slid over the loop of tube and tightened into place. The procedure was repeated with another loop of suture. Still holding the loop of tube, a segment was cut distal to the ligated tube and hemostasis was considered excellent. Both ends of the lumen of the tube could be observed.

The Valentine retractor was then lifted to the left side of the patient and the right adnexa fell into view. The procedure that had been performed on the left tube was now repeated on the right tube. Hemostasis was excellent, fimbria had been identified prior to double ligation and excision, and both ends of the lumen had been observed. *(If the adnexa do not readily fall into view, the wet JET pack is excellent to use to misplace the viscera to gain exposure.)*

All instrumentation and/or packing were removed from the peritoneum. While holding the posterior lip of the cervix upward, _____ (0-chromic) sutures were placed into the vaginal cuff and perineum in a continuous interlocking fashion along the colpotomy incision. All instrument, needle, and pack counts were correct. The patient went to the PACU in excellent condition.

# Suction dilatation and evacuation

- Cannula selection should be according to the number of weeks' gestation that the spontaneous abortion has occurred (#8 for 8 weeks' gestation). A straight cannula provides less pain, but a curved cannula is better for retroflexed or anteflexed uteri.
- Do not omit post-op meds such as:

    - RhoGAM for >12 weeks or MICRhoGAM (50 μg) if <12 weeks for patients that are Rh negative
    - consider doxycycline 100 mg po bid for a few days postoperatively to decrease risk of infection
    - Methergine, especially if >10 weeks' gestation
    - NSAIDs (nonsteroidal anti-inflammatory drugs) for post-op discomfort.

---

**Technique**

The patient was prepped and draped in the usual manner for dilatation and evacuation. A weighted speculum was placed into the vagina. Paracervical injection with 1% lidocaine was placed at 7, 9, 11, 1, 3, and 5 o'clock positions in the cervix. A straight tenaculum was used on the anterior lip of the cervix. The dilators were placed into the cervical canal until a _____ (3 mm) dilatation had been reached. A small, curved (#6, #7, #8, etc.) suction tip was then placed into the intrauterine cavity and the cavity was suctioned thoroughly in systematic fashion. Contents were retrieved and a small malleable serrated curette was used following the suction curettage. This was performed until the intrauterine cavity was felt to be smooth and empty. Bleeding was minimal and the uterus firmed up nicely. A sponge stick with a single 4 × 4 sponge was placed into the vagina and held against the cervix following the removal of all instruments. After approximately 45 seconds this was removed and the area was inspected and found to be in excellent hemostatic condition. The patient tolerated the procedure well and all instrumentation was removed and counts were correct. The patient was sent to the Recovery Room in good condition.

# Urinary incontinence procedures

## Overview

Prior to the surgical procedure, other treatments that have been tried should be mentioned in the transcription. These might be magnetic neuromodulation, pelvic power program, FemeScan, estrogens (Estring, Femring, Vagifem suppositories or creams), incontinence dish or ring, Conveen continence guard, FemAssist, FemSoft Insert, or simply Kegel's exercises or voiding diaries.

Medicines that may have been tried preoperatively, such as Ditropan, Detrol, Oxytrol patches, Vesicare, Sanctura, and Tofranil should be mentioned in the indication section of transcription.

Any tests that have been performed to help make the diagnosis for the condition that indicates the need for the procedure is good to mention prior to the surgical transcription. These could be a urine analysis, urine culture, voiding studies (micturition charts, frequency volume charts, bladder diaries, pad weighing tests, postvoid residuals, simple uroflowmetry, or pressure flow studies), urethrovesical junction mobility testing (pelvic, ultrasound, urethral pressure profile, leak point pressures, or Q-tip test), stress tests (standing cough test and/or Bonney–Marshall test), cystometry, cystometrics, levator ani electromyography, cystourethroscopy, or multichannel urodynamics.

Most specifically, when performing slings and/or periurethral injections for stress urinary incontinence (SUI) with intrinsic sphincter deficiency (ISD), it is an excellent idea to mention low MUCP (maximal urethral closure pressures) that is $\leq 20$ cmH$_2$O and/or Valsalva leak point pressure that is $>60$ cmH$_2$O.

PVR (postvoid residual) must be determined within 15 minutes of a spontaneous void. A normal PVR is 50 ml or less. However, this can be less than 100 ml if the patient has had recent urinary tract surgery. If a PVR is $>200$ ml in a patient who leaks with a cough, sneeze, or Valsalva maneuver, the diagnosis is not likely to be SUI but, rather, overflow incontinence.

Q-tip test (test for urethral hypermobility) is defined as an angle of greater than 30° either at rest or with straining.

The Marshall–Marchetti–Krantz procedure (MMK), retropubic urethropexy (Burch), and paravaginal repair have already been described (per alphabetical order) previously; therefore, they will not be presented in this chapter. Each of these procedures can be performed open or laparoscopically. If performed laparoscopically, the Capio suture-capturing device, right-sided needle holders, or German needle holders are excellent instruments for these procedures.

## SACRAL NEUROMODULATION

This procedure is the only one of its kind that can be performed for urge incontinence (detrussor incontinence or DI) refractory to appropriate conventional treatments. Most clinicians consider stress urinary incontinence to be the only type of urinary incontinence that can be treated with surgery. However, sacral nerve stimulation can be used not only for the treatment of DI but also for voiding difficulties that include dysfunctional flow with no retention (<50 ml residual), incomplete voiding or incomplete retention (>50 ml residual), or complete retention. Neuromodulation can also be used to treat urgency/frequency syndromes and chronic pelvic pain.

Neuromodulation (InterStim; Medtronic) is accomplished in two phases. The first phase is the test stimulation and the second phase is the actual surgical implantation. Each will be transcribed from actual cases.

Equipment needed is supplied in the InterStim kits.

## SACRAL NEUROMODULATION – INTERSTIM TEST STIMULATION

The patient was in the prone position, with pillows under the head and abdomen and the feet left to hang over the end of the _____ (exam or Operating Room) table to allow the surgeon to view the toes for signs of flexion. The patient was prepped and draped along the lower back and buttocks with _____ (Betadine solution) and the drapes were placed so that the sacrum and buttocks were exposed. The anatomical landmarks were marked with a standard skin marker. Xylocaine (lidocaine) 1% with sodium bicarbonate 8.4% at a 10:1 ratio was injected with a 25G, 1.5-inch needle. A _____ (3.5 or 5 inch insulated foramen needle (*similar to a spinal needle*)) was then used to test the integrity of the sacral nerves. Anal bellows and great toe flexion confirmed the location of S3; therefore, the stylet of the foramen needle was removed. The test stimulator lead was passed through the cannula of the foramen needle and placed near the appropriate sacral nerve. The foramen needle was then removed and the lead was connected to the external test stimulator for home use. The loosely coiled external portion of the lead was placed under a transparent dressing and additional gauze padding and tape was applied over the site for the patient's comfort.

Sacral X-rays with anterior, posterior, and lateral views were taken and confirmed lead position. The patient received post-op instructions on the use of the test stimulator prior to discharge home.

Voiding diaries are completed by patients from 3 to 7 days while the test stimulator is in place. At least 50% reduction in symptoms must be seen to be considered for long-term therapy. Symptoms include frequency, urgency, number of episodes of incontinence, and/or the ability to urinate without the use of an intermittent catheter. The test lead is removed in the office after completion of 3–4 days of testing. After the dressing is removed, the lead is pulled out and the site is checked for potential signs of infection. A small dressing can be placed over the site if necessary. If the patient's symptoms are at least 50% decreased and the patient desires to be a candidate for neuromodulation insertion, then fully informed consent is obtained both verbally and with videotape supplied by the manufacturer of InterStim.

---

**Pearls**

(1) It is important to ask on which side patients carry their purses, so that the IPG (implantable pulse generator) is not placed in a pouch directly under the area where the purse would rest.

(2) Patients may carry a magnet that may deactivate the device.

(3) Tips for surgical team members include the use of:

    (A) sterile water instead of saline, which is highly conductive, for irrigation

    (B) bipolar electrosurgical current near the foramen, as unipolar current could travel down the foramen

    (C) rubber-shod forceps when handling the electrodes.

---

**Specific required equipment**

(1) Basic soft tissue set (vascular forceps – Debakey, Gerald, army-navy retractors, small Richardson retractors, Weitlaner self-retaining retractors, a self-retaining retractor such as a Scott retractor, and Cobb elevators).

(2) A Balfour retractor should be available for obese patients.

(3) A set of vascular forceps must be used with rubber shods when handling the lead electrode.

(4) A 16F indwelling Foley catheter is inserted before skin prep and after positioning on the laminectomy frame.

(5) A Yankauer or Frazier suction tip, suction canister system, and electrosurgical unit.

(6) Bipolar cautery, indelible black marker, and test stimulation equipment and programmer should be available.

(7) Lead aprons or shields should be available for staff members in the event that an intraoperative X-ray is needed.

**SACRAL NEUROMODULATION – IMPLANTATION**

The patient was placed under general anesthesia using only short-acting muscle relaxants for induction so as not to inhibit nerve response when used during the procedure. After endotracheal intubation, the patient was rolled from the stretcher and placed prone on the Operating Room bed. It was insured that there was adequate padding under the bony prominences to avoid pressure on the patient's genitals and breasts. The arms and elbows were also positioned properly. The feet were positioned slightly off the end of the bed so that the toe response could be viewed easily.

A small nonsterile test stimulator dispersive pad (*supplied by the manufacturer of InterStim*) was placed on the patient's foot. This pad was connected to the test stimulator to be used during the intraoperative test stimulations. The ESU dispersive pad was placed on the patient's posterior thigh. The anatomical landmarks were marked with marker prior to prep. A catheter was then inserted. Sterile skin prep from the patient's lower back area to sacrum and perineum was then performed followed by sterile drapes, allowing exposure of the sacrum, perineum, and feet so that the pelvis and feet could be visualized during test stimulations.

A midline incision from S1 to S4 was carried out with sharp dissection. The fascia lateral to the midline was dissected using a Cobb elevator. It was divided in the direction of the incision. Peanut dissectors were also used for dissection. The paraspinal muscle fibers were sharply dissected and retracted. The sacral foramen was exposed carefully, preserving the periosteum. The S3 foramen was located by observing the anatomical landmarks.

The foramen needle was inserted at the S3 location and test stimulation was performed. The test needle was connected to the test stimulator dispersive pad on the patient's foot by a sterile cable supplied with the implant. The test foramen needle was connected by the mini-hook attached to the sterile patient cable. The test stimulator responses were monitored at this time. The needle was reinserted as needed until the desired response was obtained by observing and confirming anal bellowing and great toe flexion. *(This test stimulation also may be performed before dissection.)* After confirmation of the S3 level, the foramen needle was removed and the distal end of the electrode was inserted into the foramen using rubber-shod vascular forceps. (*A lateral X-ray may also be performed intraoperatively to confirm lead placement at this point.*)

Test stimulation was performed on each of the four electrode sites on the quadripolar connector of the lead, and responses were observed at each site. After observing _____ (anal bellowing or flexion of the great toe), the lead was anchored to the sacral bone or periosteum using _____ (nonabsorbable) suture material. The fascia of the sacral incision was then closed using interrupted _____ (polyglycolic acid) sutures. Before the fascia was completely closed, tunneling of the lead electrode was performed to the stimulator IPG site.

The stimulator IPG was placed in the _____ (flank site, lower abdomen, or upper buttock). (*Placement of the IPG in the upper buttock eliminates the need for additional position changes.*) A separate incision was made over the IPG implantation site in the upper _____ (right or left) buttock. The tunneling tool, with a plastic sheath covering it, was bent to the contour of the patient. The tip of this sharp tunneling tool was removed on the insertion end. Through the sacral incision site underneath the fascia, the tool was gently tunneled to the IPG site. After removing the tunneling tip, the metal tunneling rod was backed out, leaving the plastic tube in place. The electrode was then passed through the plastic tube to the IPG site, taking care not to introduce any blood or fluid into the plastic sheath. A laparotomy sponge was placed at both sites to keep the field dry. (*Any fluid in the lead connection site may cause shorts in the lead or IPG.*) Fluid was cleaned from the connection sites with cotton swabs as needed. The electrode was retested before connecting it to the IPG. *(If a flank or lower abdominal incision is used for the IPG site, the patient is placed in the lateral decubitus position after closure of the sacral incision site at this point in the surgery. The patient can be prepped and draped to allow exposure of the IPG and lead sites. Muscle relaxants can now be administered at this point.)*

At the IPG site, a pocket was made approximately 1 cm beneath the skin surface to ensure poper telemetry from the patient's programmer. A small plastic sleeve was placed over the electrode, which was connected to the generator using an extension cable after ensuring that all connections were dry. A plastic sleeve was slid over the connection site and secured in place with a _____ (nonabsorbable such as 2-0 silk) suture. Excess electrode wire was curled around the perimeter of the IPG. The IPG was placed in the subcutaneous pocket and tested with the programmer. *(The IPG can be deactivated after testing is completed per surgeon's preference. This allows the patient to recover from the procedure before receiving electrical stimulation.)*

Closure of the sacral fascial incision was completed with _____ suture. Subcutaneous fat was closed with _____ (absorbable ei . . . 3-0 plain) suture. Skin closure was performed using a subcutaneous technique with _____ (4-0 polyglycolic acid) suture. Full-length self-adhesive wound strips were applied after the area was clean and dry. The IPG skin site was then closed in similar manner. Sterile dressings were applied and the patient was carefully turned to a supine position. All sponge, instrument, needle, and lap counts were correct.

## SLINGS

---

### Pearls

Cullen Richardson and I used to perform sling operations using human autologous rectus fascia lata that we harvested from the patients' thighs. We eventually harvested the fascia from cadavers due to the painful graft sites on the patients' thighs. These were placed at the bladder neck. Ulmsten and colleagues eventually developed tension-free vaginal tape (TVT) in 1994 (3 years after the publication of *Surgical Transcriptions*). This mid-urethral technique results in potentially less postoperative voiding dysfunction, decreased need for postoperative catheterization, and rapid resumption of voiding. The tape recreates the support provided by the pubourethral ligaments, providing an anchoring point for the pelvic floor muscles associated with urethral closure. The TVT procedure is as effective as retropubic urethropexy and classic suburethral slings for primary treatment of SUI and may have lower complication rates.

---

Anterior intravaginal slings (anterior IVS) is a general term that covers the most commonly used methods that are performed interchangeably with the procedures TVT or TOT (transobturator tape). Therefore, an example transcription of a TVT and TOT will be given to describe the anterior IVS. The advantage of anterior IVS (TVTs or TOTs) is that these seem to be as effective and possibly more effective than the conventional repair (MMK or Burch colposuspension), without the need for an invasive abdominal or laparoscopic procedure.

There are multiple trocars that can be used with the tapes for minimally invasive sling surgery. Some examples include the TVT, Uretex, SPARC, IVS Tunnelers (USS Women's Healthcare), *Advantage, Obtryx* with curved or halo needles for transobturator mid-urethral slings *(Monarc transobturator by American Medical Systems)*, or *Lynx* for suprapubic mid-urethral sling *(Advantage, Obtryx, and Lynx are all products of Boston Scientific)*. There are also many different types of sling material from polypropylene mesh usually included in the package with the trocars. Other mesh material includes *Repliform* (Boston Scientific), *Surgipro* (Tyco US Surgical) *PelviLace, Pelvicol, or PelviTex* (Bard), *Stratasis* (Cook), *Veritas* (Synovis), and *PelviSoft* (Bard).

Four considerations for different types of slings:

(1) Monarc transobturator sling for simple primary SUI, SUI with prolapse, and potential SUI.
(2) TVT placed very loosely for recurrent SUI with leak point pressure over 60 $cmH_2O$.
(3) TVT placed with a little more tension under the urethra for patients who have recurrent SUI with leak point pressures under 60 $cmH_2O$, but who lack a complete 'drainpipe' urethra.
(4) Full fascial sling for severe ISD.

---

**Pearls**

- Try to reproduce the SUI with a cough or Valsalva maneuver if the surgery is performed under local or regional anesthesia.
- With more experience, slings are usually tied looser without losing clinical efficacy.

---

## SLINGS: TENSION-FREE VAGINAL TAPE PROCEDURE, SUBURETHRAL SLING PROCEDURE, OR ANTERIOR INTRAVAGINAL SLINGS

Some complications of TVTs reported in the literature:

- there is a 10% risk of injury to the bladder when performing TVTs
- there have been 5 deaths reported, including 4 incidents of bleeding and 1 incident of bowel injury.

## Technique

The patient was prepped and draped in the usual manner in the candy can stirrups. The bladder was completely emptied with an in-and-out catheter. Marcaine (bupivacaine) with 0.5% epinephrine was injected into the anterior vaginal mucosa along the sub mid-urethral plane and a small incision was carried out with the _____ (#11 blade) scalpel. Using the introducer, the _____ *(Advantage)* trocar was passed upward, along the urethra, penetrating the endopelvic fascia, and directed toward the ipsilateral shoulder. With gentle pressure and using the palm of the hand as a fulcrum to direct the trocar, the tip of the trocar is advanced and a slight 'give' noted as the fascia was penetrated. The handle was dropped toward the floor as the tip was directed toward the skin incision, which was made directly above the trocar tip, directly at the tented skin. Once the trocar had penetrated the puncture skin incision, the sheath was grasped with Kelly clamp and the trocar was then removed. The procedure was repeated on the opposite side. Both passes of trocars were made near the midline and close to the pubic bone so as to reduce the risk of vascular and/or neurological injuries.

Intraoperative cystourethroscopy was performed at this point to confirm bladder integrity. *(If unintentional bladder perforation is noted, it is typically very small and located near the dome of the bladder – safe distance from the urethral orifices. The trocar is withdrawn and reintroduced and a catheter is all that is required postoperatively for a few days. The perforation should heal spontaneously by that time with an indwelling catheter).* Once correct trocar placement was confirmed, the sleeves were advanced upward bilaterally. This was performed until the sling was in place beneath the mid-urethra. Correct tension was adjusted with external bladder Crede maneuver. *(If the patient is awake and under spinal or epidural anesthesia, correct tension can be made by having the patient cough.)* Tension was performed at a standard volume of approximately 300 ml. The sleeves were removed and excess sling was cut just beneath the skin after tension had been adjusted. Both small skin incisions were closed with a _____ (5-0 subcuticular or one 2-0 nylon) stitch. The suburethral vaginal incision was closed with _____ (2-0 chromic or 2-0 Vicryl). All sponge, needle, and instrument counts were correct. The patient went to the PACU in good condition.

## SLINGS: TRANSOBTURATOR TAPE PROCEDURE

### Considerations

- There is less chance of bladder injury with this procedure.
- There have been some reports of increased pain in the genital-femoral folds.
- There are some safety issues still being studied regarding the close proximity of the obturator nerve and vessels (4.4 cm from obturator vessel and 2.2–2.8 cm from the obturator nerve).
- There is less urinary retention at post op day one (13.3 % TOT vs 25.8% TVT).
- There is less operative time (TOT = 15 minutes versus TVT = 27 minutes).
- This procedure is performed outside to inside versus inside to outside.
- Caldera Medical supplies the T-sling with Centrasorb (a large-pore monofilament polypropylene). There are multiple reusable introducers in this system so that the TOT can be performed via the vaginal or suprapubic approach with the curved introducers or the transobturator approach with the helical, inside-out, or hook introducers.

### Technique

The patient was prepped and draped in the usual manner, with special attention to the inferior pubic ramus and vaginal operative sites. Marcaine with 0.5% epinephrine was injected into the vaginal wall in preparation for the incision. A small anterior vaginal wall incision was carried out and dissection was made bilaterally to the interior portion of the inferior pubic ramus. A vertical skin incision was carried out large enough to insert the _____ (curved) needle tip just lateral to the edge of the inferior pubic ramus at the junction where the inferior pubic ramus and adductor longus muscle meet. The same was performed on the contralateral side. The _____ (curved) needle device handle was grasped and the needle inserted through one skin incision, piercing through the obturator muscle and obturator membrane. The handle was turned at a 45° angle medial towards the lateral dissection of the vaginal incision, placing the fingertip on the distal end of the needle. The distal end of the needle was guided around the inferior pubic ramus through the vaginal incision, maintaining contact with the finger.

Loop engagement was made at the distal end of the needle. The needle was pulled out through the skin incision, making sure the mesh assembly was not twisted and that it was flat under the urethra, with the blue centering tab positioned suburethrally, facing outward. The association loop was removed from the needle. The same procedure for inserting the needle and engaging the loop was performed on the contralateral side, making certain to stay just lateral to the edge of the inferior pubic ramus.

Cystoscopy was performed to insure the integrity of the bladder. Once the bladder was noted to have no unintentional injury, the mesh/sleeve assembly was pulled outwards on the dilators so that the blue centering tab was centered below the urethra. Tension was adjusted by bladder Crede maneuver with 300 ml of sterile water in the bladder. The blue centering tab was grasped and the tab was cut through the center of the punch hole, ensuring that both halves of the blue tab were completely removed from the vaginal canal. The dilators were pulled outward to remove the sleeves, leaving the mesh in place. The tension was again verified and adjustments made as necessary. The skin incisions were gently pushed downward and the distal ends of the mesh were cut, confirming that the ends retracted into the skin incisions. The skin incisions were closed with _____ (5-0 Vicryl subcuticular or 2-0 or 3-0 nylon) sutures. The vaginal incisions were closed with _____ (2-0 Vicryl). All sponge, instruments, and needle counts were correct. The patient went to the PACU in excellent condition.

## SLINGS: TRANSVAGINAL SUBURETHRAL SLING PROCEDURE USING THE 'INFLUENCE' DRILL

Occasionally, some clinicians believe that a urethra that has an increased hypermobility can be immobilized better with a *transvaginal suburethral sling procedure using the posterior pubic drilling of titanium screws*. This procedure may also have an advantage in patients with previous urinary incontinent procedures. The downside is the increased risk of osteitis of the pubic bone. Osteitis is very rare; however, following antiseptic procedures (given below) can even decrease this risk further.

### Technique

The patient was prepped and draped in the dorsal lithotomy position with Betadine solution. An injection of approximately ——— (10 ml) of Marcaine 0.5% with epinephrine was carried out along the midline of the anterior vagina. A midline incision was performed through the vaginal mucosa, extending from the apex of the vagina to the urethral meatus. Flaps of the vagina were dissected laterally with sharp dissection. Bleeding was controlled using electrocautery and _____ (2-0 Vicryl detachable on a Uro-6 needle) suture.

The periurethral and perivesical fascia were immobilized widely by blunt finger dissection using a single layer of gauze sponge. Entering into the white-appearing, avascular plane just beneath the vaginal mucosa and facilitating fascial mobilization, the dissection was carried out to the most lateral aspect of the urethra and bladder base. From a point less than 1 cm from the urethral meatus, successful vertical mattress sutures were made in the periurethral fascia. Bites were taken on each side of the urethra at points of bleeding.

With the bladder still mobilized and exposed, especially at the bladder base and prior to closing under this, the _____ *(PelviSoft, Repliform, etc.)* transvaginal allograft was picked up with forceps out of the _____ (bacitracin, Neosporin, penicillin, ampicillin, etc.) antibiotic solution. This was inspected and assured that the allograft was of the correct size and shape. This was placed back into the solution to soak for 15–20 minutes.

A catheter was placed back into the urethra. After a modified anterior repair was performed, thus reducing any cystocele, a titanium bone screw with attached Prolene suture was placed in the *Influence* drill (American Medical). The drill with screw tip was placed behind the pubic bone, lateral to the urethra at the bladder neck. The bone screw was in place and pulled up firmly, confirming the position of the instrument. The bone screw was drilled into the posterior aspect of the pubic bone until the sound of the drill indicated that the drill had firmly placed the screw properly in the bone. The same was done on the contralateral side of the urethra. As the instrument was pulled out on each side, the Prolene suture was exposed. A firm pull on the Prolene suture confirmed secure placement of the titanium screws on both sides of the urethra.

Cystoscopy was performed to insure the integrity of the urethra and ureteral orifices. There were no injuries noted throughout the bladder.

The graft was obtained from the antibiotic solution. An 18-gauge needle was placed through the edges of the allograft and the Prolene suture was placed through the bore of the needle and used to thread the Prolene suture back through the allograft. Using a smooth curette to push the Prolene suture up into position, confirmation was made that the graft was not too tense. The sling was then secured into position by tying the Prolene sutures, making sure there was no excess tension. Irrigation was performed with _____. The anterior and posterior edges of the graft were sutured into the periurethral fascia with _____ (#2-0 Vicryl) suture on a small URO-6 needle. At the urethrovesical junction, the peri-urethral fascia was drawn carefully from its most lateral margin to add additional support to the posterior urethra. Excess Prolene suture that was noted to be protruding from the knots in the allograft was then melted with an ophthalmological cautery until the ends were blunt.

Any excess vaginal mucosa was excised and the margins of the vagina were approximated in the midline using an interupted _____ (2-0 Vicryl) suture. The bladder was emptied and then 500 ml of normal sterile saline was injected into the bladder via a catheter. The catheter was clamped and, at this point, a suprapubic catheter was placed at two fingerbreadths above the symphysis pubis until fluid could be drawn up into a syringe and noted to be clear. The suprapubic catheter was sutured into place with _____ (3-0 nylon) and plugged *(or can be attached to a Foley bag to gravity if bladder training will not take place until the next day)*. All sponge, needle, and instrument counts were correct. The patient went to the PACU in good condition.

## POSTERIOR INTRAVAGINAL SLINGS

Although this is a sling procedure, the indication is for vaginal prolapse rather than urinary incontinence; therefore, it can be found in alphabetical order in this book.

## PERIURETHRAL BULKING PROCEDURE

The periurethral bulking agents most commonly used are Contigen (Bard), which is essentially a collagen product, and Durasphere (Carbon Medical Technologies), which comprises microscopic carbon beads. The indication for this procedure is intrinsic sphincter deficiency. This procedure is an excellent choice for patients at higher risk for more invasive sling procedures for the same indication. The author's product of choice at this time is Durasphere for several advantageous reasons:

(1)  since this substance is inert, there is no need for allergy testing
(2)  it is permanent; therefore, one does not need to concern oneself about repeat treatments every year or two as one would with the dissolving of a collagen product
(3)  it is radiopaque and therefore one can evaluate the placement around the urethrovesical junction with X-ray if necessary.

Although these procedures can be performed in an office setting, the author has found it more advantageous to use the outpatient Operating Room for providing MAC and/or general or regional anesthesia in these usually older patients.

### Technique

The patient was prepped and draped in the routine manner. The cystoscope was advanced into the bladder and backed up to the UV junction. While the examination demonstrated the UV junction, the fingertip was placed at the site of the cystoscope, which was at the junction of the urethral meatus, and then the cystoscope was removed. The length from the urethral meatus to the UV junction was measured. Marcaine 0.5% with epinephrine was inserted at the 5 and 7 o'clock positions, approximately 1–2 cm from the urethral meatus. *(There are bilateral indentations just inside the vaginal introitus at these positions of injection.)* The needle was pushed back along the length of the urethra to the sides of the UV junction. Approximately 10 ml of anesthetic was injected into each site. A Durasphere syringe with a 45° curved needle was then injected at the 5 o'clock position while watching the bulging at the UV junction. The same procedure was repeated at the 7 o'clock position. The injections were repeated _____ times, with _____ *(usually 4–6)* Durasphere syringes until examination demonstrated excellent bulking and closing of the UV junction. Once all the syringes had been removed, a small sponge was held with moderate pressure for approximately 45 seconds on the injection sites until there was excellent hemostasis. All needle, instruments, and sponge counts were correct. The patient left the _____ *(Examining Room or Operating Room)* in excellent condition.

# Vulvectomy

## Technique

After the patient has been properly prepped and draped, the groin dissection was started with two teams. The groin incision was extended in an arcuate fashion from each anterior iliac superior crest, passing 2 cm above the symphysis and inguinal ligament. The butterfly vulvar incision includes the skin over the region of the fossa ovalis. The incision was extended inferiorly along the lateral aspect of the labia majora so as to remove all of the perineal body and tissue around the superior aspect of the anus. The skin and subcutaneous fat, including Camper's and Scarpa's fascia, were dissected to remove the superficial lymphatic channels and to avoid necrosis of skin margins. The incision was modified along the _____ (labiocrural folds, clitoris, or wherever the tumor is near) so that the incision extended for at least 2 cm beyond the tumor margins.

The lateral incision was extended to the fascia lata. The superior incision was made so as to remove all the lymphatic and areolar tissue down to the oponeurosis of the external oblique and anterior rectus fascia. Dissection was continued from the lateral aspect of the inguinal ligament to the region of the mons pubis.

The femoral sheath was incised along the medial margin of the sartorius muscle and along the lateral side of the artery. The femoral artery was palpated for identification and the femoral nerve was identified adjacent to it. The cribriform fascia was completely dissected off the artery and the external pudendal artery was carefully identified and ligated. The proximal end of the saphenous vein was transfixed and doubly ligated with _____ suture. The femoral sheath was dissected medially as an en bloc procedure.

The distal segment of the saphenous vein was ligated and excised as the dissection was continued toward the inner thigh.

Vulvar dissection was continued to include the perineal skin along the lateral side of the anus, a major portion of each labia, and along the periosteum of the symphysis at the level of the fascia of the deep musculature of the urogenital diaphragm. Thus, the bulbocavernosus, ischiocavernosus, and superficial transverse perinei muscles were removed.

The internal pudendal vessels were ligated with _____ suture as these were identified emerging from Alcock's canal at the 4 and 8 o'clock positions.

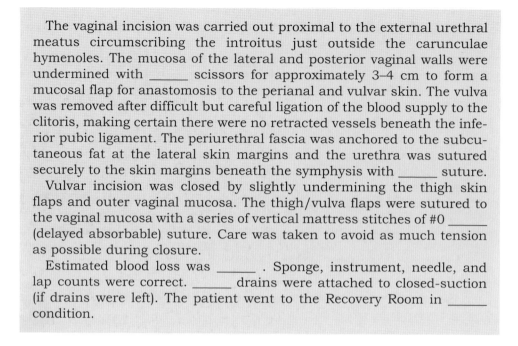

The vaginal incision was carried out proximal to the external urethral meatus circumscribing the introitus just outside the carunculae hymenoles. The mucosa of the lateral and posterior vaginal walls were undermined with _____ scissors for approximately 3–4 cm to form a mucosal flap for anastomosis to the perianal and vulvar skin. The vulva was removed after difficult but careful ligation of the blood supply to the clitoris, making certain there were no retracted vessels beneath the inferior pubic ligament. The periurethral fascia was anchored to the subcutaneous fat at the lateral skin margins and the urethra was sutured securely to the skin margins beneath the symphysis with _____ suture.

Vulvar incision was closed by slightly undermining the thigh skin flaps and outer vaginal mucosa. The thigh/vulva flaps were sutured to the vaginal mucosa with a series of vertical mattress stitches of #0 _____ (delayed absorbable) suture. Care was taken to avoid as much tension as possible during closure.

Estimated blood loss was _____ . Sponge, instrument, needle, and lap counts were correct. _____ drains were attached to closed-suction (if drains were left). The patient went to the Recovery Room in _____ condition.

**Author's note**

Transcribe inguinal node dissection if performed and include description of drain placements if necessary.

Remember that if tumor is near the urethra or along the medial aspect of the labia minora – the outer one-third of the urethra should be removed and described. If cystourethrocele is present, plication and retropubic elevation of the urethrovesical angle would be necessary to avoid urinary incontinence and should also be described.

Each vulvectomy must be individualized according to whether simple, radical, separate incisions, unilateral or even exenteration would need to be performed depending on depth of stromal invasion, tumor size, and location of tumor. 5500 rads of midpelvic megavoltage pelvic irradiation might be recommended versus further deep node dissection and transcription depending upon evidence of groin metastasis. The author presently refers this surgery to oncology services secondary to lack of facilities and consultation in his rural area. This procedure is included for the benefit of residents and interns.